'The Plant-Based Diet Revolution is precisely what the world needs right now. Between these covers you'll find clear and easy-to-digest explanations of the science, beautiful whole-food recipes, and the step-by-step plan you need to harness the power of the food on your plate and truly revolutionise your health and wellbeing.'
Julieanna Hever, MS RD CPT, Plant-Based Dietitian, author of Plant-Based Nutrition (Idiot's Guide) and The Vegiterranean Diet

'Get ready, because this book is going to change your life in so many positive ways! Dr Alan Desmond makes a powerful argument for plant-based food, and he makes it easy to shift in that direction with well-researched advice and delicious recipes. Enjoy the journey; it's a deeply gratifying one!'
Kathy Freston, New York Times best-selling author of Quantum Wellness, The Lean and Clean Protein

'The status quo is beyond unsustainable… it's actually killing us. Now is the time for a shake-up to restore our health and get us back to thriving once more. Dr Alan Desmond's The Plant-Based Diet Revolution will introduce a new era of delicious food that promotes a healthy mind, body and gut. Long live – and live long in – the revolution!'
Dr Will Bulsiewicz, MSCI, New York Times bestselling author of Fiber Fueled

'Think you can't get stronger, faster and reach new athletic heights on plants? Think again. This book itself is a revolution in the evolution of health. Be prepared to have your mind blown.'
Dotsie Bausch, track cyclist, Olympic medal winner, eight times US National Champion and star of The Gamechangers

'This book is fantastic. We love the recipes and secretly wish that we'd written them ourselves!'
Stephen and David Flynn, The Happy Pear.

'The Plant-Based Diet Revolution has all the stepping stones you need to confidently improve your eating habits and health. With sound scientific information from one of the world's leading experts, ingenious tips, and delicious recipes, you have everything you need to change your health and life for the better. Authoritative, practical, and beautifully laid out.'
Dr Neal D. Barnard, FACC, Adjunct Professor, George Washington University School of Medicine and President of the Physicians Committee for Responsible Medicine

'With The Plant-Based Diet Revolution, Dr Alan Desmond has given us a tapestry of delicious plant-based food that can protect us from disease and provide us with optimal health and longevity.'
Dr Caldwell B. Esselstyn, Jr, author of Prevent and Reverse Heart Disease

'Like the author himself, The Plant-Based Diet Revolution is a bright, informative and unfailingly enthusiastic guide to the healthful, sumptuous and sustainable world of plant-based cuisine. This is the book I wish I had written on this important topic and I'll be recommending The Plant-Based Diet Revolution to my many patients who are serious about eating their way to better health.'
Dr Michael Klaper, Program Director of Moving Medicine Forward and author of Vegan Nutrition Pure and Simple

'Never before has the food that we put on our plates been more important. Dr Alan is a wealth of knowledge and in The Plant-Based Diet Revolution he provides you with all the tools you need to eat for a healthier and happier life.'
Dr Rupy Aujla, NHS Doctor and author of The Doctor's Kitchen

'The Doc and I are on the same mission: to give people the knowledge and tools they'll need to embrace plant-based eating more easily! This book is awesome, laying out the science that clears up any confusion for those thinking about making the switch to plants. It's a gateway to better meals and, of course, better health as a result. My advice is to join the plant-based diet revolution today!'
Derek Sarno, chef, Director of Plant-Based Innovation at Tesco, co-founder of Wicked Kitchen and co-author of The Wicked Healthy Cookbook

'The food we choose on a daily basis has a more powerful impact on our lives than many of us realise. This book provides everything you need to discover the compelling science and experience the astonishing results of plant-based eating for yourself. Come and join the plant-based diet revolution and discover what it could do for you.'
Rosie Martin, Registered Dietician and Advisory Board Member, Plant-Based Health Professionals UK

'The Plant-Based Diet Revolution is an absolutely stunning book. I have not seen a more comprehensive, insightful and engaging plant-based guidebook. The recipes are accompanied by gorgeous photos that would tempt anyone – plant-leaning or otherwise. This book makes an enormous contribution to the world of lifestyle medicine!'
Brenda Davis, Registered Dietitian, plant-based pioneer, co-author of Nourish: the Definitive Nutrition Guide for Plant-Based Families

'A truly wonderful read. Dr Alan has taken complex nutritional science and made it understandable to everyone. The recipes are so eclectic, colourful and varied but yet attainable to everyone, no matter what your budget or kitchen skills. All this coming from a doctor; yes, please! Take the Doctor's orders and join the plant-based diet revolution today.'
Tanya O'Callaghan, professional rock musician and co-host of Highway to Health

'The Plant-Based Diet Revolution provides you with the information you need to make the transition to a healthy plant-based diet. Easy to understand, yet evidence-based, it also details Dr Desmond's hands-on experience as a Gastroenterologist and his use of 'food as medicine' to help his patients heal. Once read, you will be left with no doubt that a plant-based diet is right for you!'
Dr Shireen Kassam, Consultant Haematologist and Certified Lifestyle Medicine Physician

'The food in The Plant-Based Diet Revolution is bursting with colour and flavour. Dr Alan Desmond's solid, evidence-based approach is paired with vibrant and nutritious recipes that are easy to follow for busy people.'
Dr Rajiv Bajekal, FRCS Orth, Consultant Spinal Surgeon and Lifestyle Medicine Physician

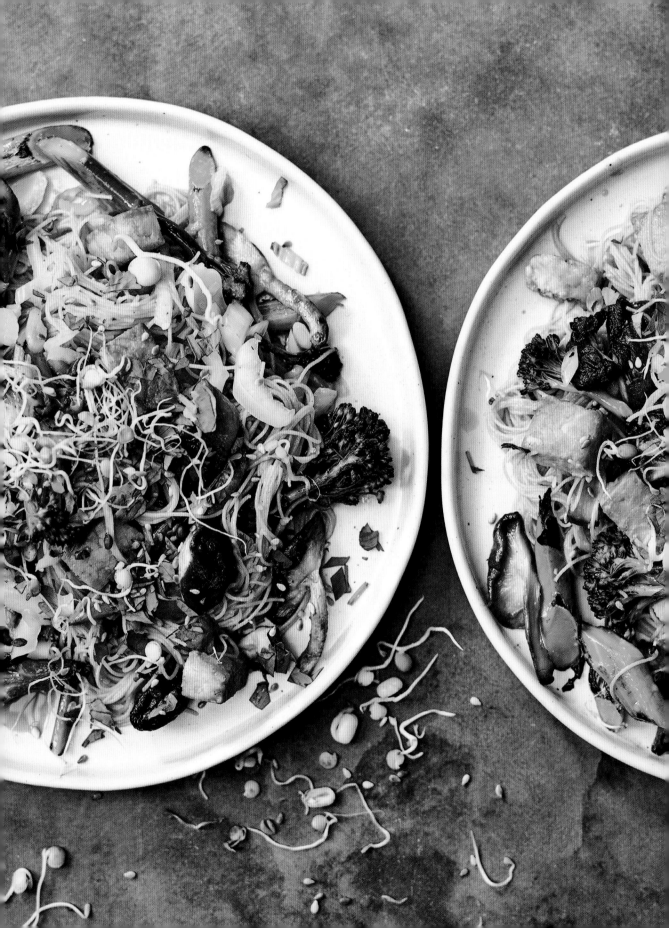

THE PLANT-BASED DIET REVOLUTION

28 days to a happier gut and a healthier you

DR ALAN DESMOND

WITH 80 SIMPLE VEGAN RECIPES BY BOB ANDREW

Foreword by THE HAPPY PEAR

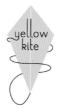

yellow kite

Diet (noun): The food that a person or animal regularly eats.

Collins English Dictionary

'We know enough. We truly know enough to make a whole-food, plant-based diet our number one recommendation for the prevention and treatment of so many chronic diseases.'

Brenda Davis, Registered Dietitian

For Hannah, Rebecca, Naomi and Ethan. I love you to the moon — and back.

First published in Great Britain in 2021 by Yellow Kite
An imprint of Hodder & Stoughton
An Hachette UK company

1

Copyright © 2021 Dr Alan Desmond, recipes Bob Andrew
Photography copyright © Dan Jones

Photography on pages 11, 13, 15, 19, 21, 25, 27, 32, 47, 49, 51, 54, 57, 61, 198 and 201 © Shutterstock.com
Photo on page 6 © The Happy Pear
Reproduced with permission

The right of Dr Alan Desmond and Bob Andrew to be identified as the Authors of the Work has been asserted by them in accordance with the Copyright, Designs and Patents Act 1988.

A CIP catalogue record for this title is available from the British Library

Hardback ISBN 978 1 529 30868 6
eBook ISBN 978 1 529 31017 7

Editorial Director: Nicky Ross
Project Editor: Sophie Elletson
Design: Louise Leffler
Photography: Dan Jones
Food Stylist: Samantha Dixon
Props Stylist: Charlie Phillips

Colour origination by Altaimage
Printed and bound in Italy by L.E.G.O. SpA

Hodder & Stoughton policy is to use papers that are natural, renewable and recyclable products and made from wood grown in sustainable forests. The logging and manufacturing processes are expected to conform to the environmental regulations of the country of origin.

Yellow Kite Books
Hodder & Stoughton Ltd
Carmelite House
50 Victoria Embankment
London
EC4Y 0DZ

www.yellowkitebooks.co.uk
www.hodder.co.uk

CONTENTS

Foreword by Steven and David Flynn of The Happy Pear **06**
Introduction: Join the revolution! **07**

PART 1: THE POWER OF THE FOOD ON YOUR PLATE
Why food really matters **09**
The whole-food, plant-based approach **14**
Doctor's orders: ten prescriptions for better health **22**

PART 2: UNLOCKING THE PLANT-BASED ADVANTAGE
Healthy gut **29**
Healthy heart **38**
Healthy body **44**
Healthy mind **52**
Lessons from the pandemic **57**

PART 3: RECIPES FOR THE REVOLUTION
Getting the basics right **59**
Breakfasts **62**
Lighter meals **84**
Main meals **122**
Sweet treats **174**

PART 4: THE 28-DAY REVOLUTION
Preparing for the revolution **195**
Start the revolution: meal plans & cooking guide **200**
Celebrate success and move forward **210**

PART 5: QUESTIONS, ANSWERS AND RECOMMENDED RESOURCES
Plant-based Q&A **212**
The A to Z of plants in your kitchen **215**
Recommended resources **218**

Index **219**
Acknowledgements **224**

Foreword

by Steven and David Flynn of The Happy Pear

Dr Alan Desmond has taught us and our community so much about how the food we eat affects our health and happiness. This book is fantastic! Not only does it explain the science behind why you should eat your veggies, it also shows you how to do it. We love the recipes, and secretly wish we'd written them ourselves!

We've been eating a plant-based diet for almost twenty years. As identical twin brothers, it started out as a competition to find out who could be the healthier twin! Changing our approach to food really transformed our lives. Having experienced the benefits for ourselves, we set about spreading the word. Through our Happy Pear restaurants, our best-selling cookery books, our successful YouTube channel and our online courses, we've helped thousands of people to eat more veg. The incredible benefits of a diet that's packed with beans, greens, wholegrains, fruits and veggies are now recognised by mainstream medicine, and in the last few years we've been delighted to watch as more people than ever decide to move towards a plant-based diet.

We're delighted that you've decided to join the Plant-Based Diet Revolution, and we know that you're in good hands with Dr Alan.

Enjoy!

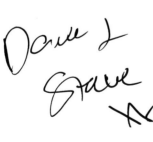

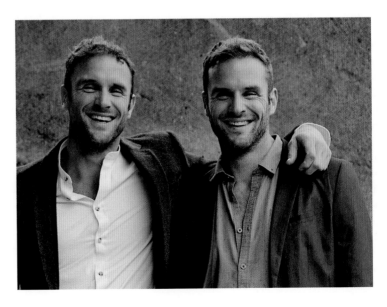

INTRODUCTION
JOIN THE REVOLUTION!

As a doctor I've explained a new diagnosis to thousands of patients. My specialty is Gastroenterology – the diagnosis and treatment of digestive health problems. Faced with a new illness, every patient soon asks me about food: 'Is there anything that I should or shouldn't eat?' I view it as my professional duty to have evidence-based answers to this question. We each know intuitively that food can play a vital role in helping us to improve our health, optimise our quality of life and even help us to heal and recover from illness. The scientific evidence shows that this is absolutely true. Food is medicine. To maximise your chances of health right now and into the future, to reduce your risk of chronic illness and to add healthy years to your life, you must start with the food on your plate. This book cuts through the diet confusion by clearly explaining the science and giving you the practical skills that you need to make healthier choices every time you eat.

Doctors are trained to examine the scientific research and then make evidence-based recommendations to their patients. After years spent examining the research on diet, nutrition and health, I am convinced that the more plants and the fewer processed foods on our plates the better. The logical conclusion? A whole-food, plant-based diet. A diet that is built from the nutritious foods that humans have thrived on for centuries – fruits, vegetables, beans, wholegrains, nuts and seeds – can produce incredible benefits in both preventing chronic disease and restoring true health. Whether we are aiming to prevent or treat heart disease, obesity, type 2 diabetes, irritable bowel syndrome, Crohn's disease, digestive cancers, or any of the diseases that have become so common in the 21st century, a plant-based diet has something to offer.

I now start conversations with my patients by asking about the foods they eat each day. Evidence-based dietary advice helps my patients to get the best possible outcomes. I am privileged to work alongside a team of highly qualified dietitians who work to the same principles. This approach has revolutionised my clinical practice and the lives of many of my patients. By putting more plants on their plates, I have seen individuals of all ages improve both their gut health and overall health, lose weight, improve their mood and even reverse long-term illness.

Supporting patients in making healthy dietary changes has become just as important as the procedures I perform and the medications I prescribe. Inspired by my patients, I decided that I had to take this message to a wider audience. Through speaking engagements at home and abroad, academic publications, presentations at scientific conferences, lectures to doctors in training, interviews with journalists and even through my social media accounts, I have embraced every opportunity to share their inspiring stories and to explain the science that continues to shape my practice.

Within this book you'll find the knowledge and practical skills that you need to bring the same evidence-based approach into your kitchen and onto your plate. You'll learn about the true power of the food on your plate, my ten prescriptions for better health and the incredible role that our gut microbes play in helping us to improve every aspect of our health and well-being, and you'll read inspiring stories from people just like you who've benefited from making the switch to a plant-based diet. I've teamed up with my good friend and talented chef Bob Andrew to turn the science of healthy eating into delicious plant-based recipes for you to enjoy every day. Once you've experienced how satisfying dishes like Quick banana and blueberry pancakes, Loaded sweet potato with jerk black beans & peppers, or Hearty Bolognese with squash & rosemary polenta are, I hope that you'll push things to the next level and commit to 28 days thriving on plants. 'The 28-Day Revolution' provides the shopping lists, practical tips and dietitian-approved meal plans you'll need to experience the benefits of a completely plant-based diet for yourself.

Thank you for making your health a priority. Let's start your revolution!

NOTE: The text includes stories of patients I have treated at my clinic. Names and some details have been changed to protect anonymity. Where needed, permission has been given. I have provided references for the scientific papers that inform my approach to nutrition and human health. I encourage you to read these for yourself. You can access the full list of references by visiting alandesmond.com/revolution

PART ONE

THE POWER OF THE FOOD ON YOUR PLATE

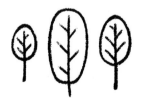

WHY FOOD REALLY MATTERS

Becoming a doctor takes a long time. I entered medical school in 1995 and qualified as a doctor in 2001. By 2003 I had two years of clinical practice behind me and was working at a busy university hospital. Life as a junior hospital doctor meant regularly clocking up more than 100 hours on duty per week. Thirty-six-hour shifts without protected breaks were the norm. During that busy time, I had my first stint in gastroenterology, as a junior member of a team of doctors and other health professionals caring for patients with serious digestive problems. I quickly realised that this was the speciality I wanted to dedicate my professional career to. I would go on to complete another nine years of training before qualifying as a consultant gastroenterologist in 2012.

Back in 2003, one of the patients on our gastroenterology ward was a 19-year-old man with a new diagnosis of Crohn's disease, a condition that causes inflammation within the gut and its lining. For both doctor and patient, this condition can be exceedingly difficult to manage. (1, 2) After two days of receiving strong steroid medications to reduce the inflammation, our patient was doing quite well. We reassured him that the treatment was working. The likelihood of needing surgery in the short term was low. We planned to start a new immune-suppressing medication within days and soon he would be able to eat normally again. Then came the questions: 'What about food, doctor? Is there anything that I should eat? Are there any foods I should avoid?' The consultant's answer surprised him: 'It doesn't matter. Eat whatever you feel like. Calories are important for healing. Do you like McDonald's? Ask your mum to bring some in.' That answer reflected the mainstream thinking at the time. Calories were just calories.

As I progressed through my medical training, it struck me that every patient faced with a new diagnosis – whether it be Crohn's disease, colitis, irritable bowel syndrome or any other gut problem – asked me the same question: 'What about food?' Were there any things they should eat or avoid in order to feel better and improve their outlook in the months and years to come? Increasingly, I found the standard answer – 'Calories are calories regardless of the source' – just didn't make any sense. This is what prompted me to seek out evidence-based answers to my patients' questions about food. I would find them in the same medical journals and textbooks that taught me the most recent procedural techniques and the latest advances in drug therapies. As I discovered, the science is clear: when it comes to human health, food really matters.

THE RISE OF THE STANDARD WESTERN DIET

Doctors have known that food is tightly linked to health and disease since the dawn of modern medicine. In the fifth century BC, the Greek physician Hippocrates taught his students that diet was the most powerful tool of all in maintaining health and treating disease. (3) In the 20th century the importance of the food on our plates became obvious as we saw that dramatic increases in obesity, heart disease and type 2 diabetes were closely linked to the rise of the Standard Western Diet, a new way of eating that depends largely on animal products and industrially produced foods. (4) These trends continued into the 21st century. We now consume more meat, more dairy and more highly processed 'junk' foods than ever before in human history. Many of us have all but stopped eating the nutritious foods that humans have thrived on for centuries – fruits, vegetables, beans, wholegrains, nuts and seeds.

For our ancient ancestors, life was a daily struggle for calories. In times of almost constant malnutrition, food was probably defined as any edible substance, animal or vegetable, that they could get their hands on. A long and happy retirement was never on the cards; their goal was simply to live long enough to pass on their genes and ensure the survival of their family and the tribe. The rare opportunity to eat a calorie-dense meal packed with sugar, salt, fat or animal protein could not be passed up. At a basic level, humans are still wired to seek out calorie-dense foods. The food industry knows this and profits by designing products that are just that and more. Menu options such as 'bacon double cheeseburger with fries' and 'sugar-coated cinnamon donut sticks' have been carefully crafted to be almost irresistible to our primitive brains.

The drive for calorie-rich foods that helped our ancient ancestors to survive into early adulthood has been used to corrupt our approach to food, leading to a surge in obesity and poor health. Globally, 255 million healthy years of life are lost to the Standard Western Diet each year. (5) Most people, if asked to write down a list of the leading causes of disease in the UK, would probably include things such as lack of exercise, air pollution and smoking. Those issues are important, and they do make the list. But the food we eat beats them all. Thanks to our Standard Western Diet, food is now responsible for causing more disease and disability in the UK than alcohol and drug abuse combined. (6) In the United States, food has overtaken cigarettes to become the number one cause of poor health and premature death. (7)

WHAT SHOULD I EAT?

As rates of obesity, heart disease and type 2 diabetes have continued to soar, 'What should I eat?' has become one of the most important questions of the 21st century. The prestigious medical journal the *Lancet* recently asked a high-powered team of experts from around the globe to find the answer. Having analysed decades of scientific research on health and nutrition, here's how their EAT-Lancet report (8) describes a healthy diet for everyone: 'A planetary health plate should consist by volume of approximately half a plate of vegetables and fruits; the other half should consist of primarily wholegrains, plant protein sources, unsaturated plant oils, and (optionally) modest amounts of animal sources of protein.'

You might find it surprising to learn that meat, dairy and eggs are not needed for a healthy diet. If you do choose to include these foods, the evidence shows that the safest amounts to eat are very small: just 29g of chicken, 28g of fish or 13g of egg per day. When a medium egg weighs in at 50g, it hardly seems worth cracking one open! The expert advice on red meat is especially clear. The more you eat, the greater your chances of poor health. The experts who compiled the EAT-Lancet report gave the following advice on red meat: 'Optimal intake may be zero grams per day, especially if replaced by plant sources of protein.'

The science clearly shows that a global shift to a plant-based diet would have major benefits, preventing an estimated 11.6 million adult deaths per year. (8) In recent years we have seen the meat, dairy and egg sections removed from national healthy eating guidelines. (9) A plant-based diet has been endorsed as a healthy choice by the British Dietetic Association, the American Academy of Nutrition and Dietetics, the Canadian healthy eating guidelines, the American Cancer Society, the World Health Organisation, the American College of Lifestyle Medicine and numerous other organisations. (10-15) The plant-based diet revolution has truly entered the mainstream!

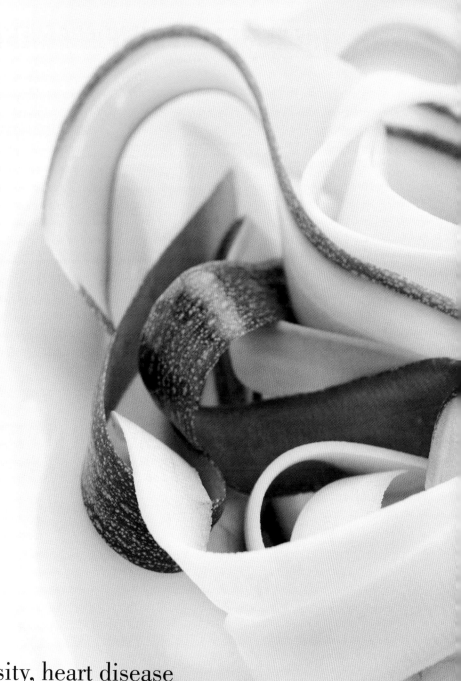

As rates of obesity, heart disease
and type 2 diabetes continue to soar,
'What should I eat?' has become one
of the most important questions
of the 21st century.

THE OPPOSITE OF HEALTHY

The science is clear: we can live longer and healthier lives by minimising our intake of processed foods, added oils and animal products, and by choosing healthy plant-based options first. Knowing this, it's astounding how much of the harmful – and how little of the beneficial – foods we eat. For most people in the industrialised world, food has become the opposite of healthy. In the US the 'unhealthy three' – processed foods, added oils and animal products – account for 60% of all calories consumed, while fruits, vegetables and legumes make up just 9%. Despite the fact that wholegrains are hugely beneficial to human health, the vast majority of the grains eaten today are the highly processed refined grains found in cakes, mass-produced breads and pastries. (16, 17) The nation that invented the Standard Western Diet and where food is the number one cause of preventable death is also a world leader in eating meat. US meat consumption has been on the rise for decades and shows no signs of slowing. (18) In 2018, the US Department of Agriculture announced that the US had hit 'peak meat', with an estimated 100kg (220lb) of red meat and poultry consumed per person that year. (19)

A similar disease-promoting approach to food is now a truly global phenomenon. When it comes to fruits and vegetables, fewer than one in three British adults make it to the modest five-a-day target. Britain is behind the US on annual meat consumption, but still manages 83kg (183lb) per person. Our current dietary choices mean that 12% of all calories come from the unhealthy saturated fats found primarily in meat, dairy and processed foods. (20) One in three European adults does not consume fruits and vegetables on a daily basis. (21) Wholegrains, beans, greens and legumes have been pushed out in favour of fast food, take-aways, processed meat pies and white bread bacon butties! Most of the meals we eat are built from the foods that are making us ill. To quote Public Health England's chief expert on diet and nutrition: 'Poor diets are all too common in this country and, along with obesity, are now one of the leading causes of ... cancer, heart disease and type 2 diabetes. It's clear from these data that the nation's diet needs an overhaul.' (22) I couldn't agree more.

THE POWER OF A HEALTHIER APPROACH TO FOOD

Although the Standard Western Diet appears to have taken over the world, it is possible to find people with a healthier approach to food. In 2014 a team of Belgian researchers set out to find them. (23) They collected detailed food diaries from almost 1,500 adults and classified them into four dietary groups: vegan (completely plant-based), vegetarian (plant-based plus eggs or dairy), pescatarian (vegetarian plus fish) and omnivores (everything, including meat). They rated everybody's diet for healthy content using two established research tools: the Healthy Eating Index (HEI), which gives points for making food choices in keeping with the US Department of Agriculture Food Pyramid; and the Mediterranean Diet Score (MDS), which scores higher the more your diet complies with guidelines for a healthy Mediterranean diet.

On both rating systems, those who maintained a completely plant-based diet scored the healthiest of all four groups. Omnivores fared badly, getting the lowest scores. The researchers noted that plant-based eaters benefited from several advantages over omnivores: lower total calories, lower saturated fat and lower sodium intake. They also had a higher intake of whole fruits, beans and greens, and were the least likely of all four groups to be obese. Those eating a completely plant-based diet did consume slightly less protein, but with an average 82g of plant-based protein per day, they were still getting more than enough. The researchers concluded: 'Estimating the overall diet quality based on different aspects of healthful dietary models indicated consistently the vegan diet as the most healthy.'

This healthier approach to food is certainly worth the effort. When European researchers analysed diet quality and health outcomes in 1.6 million people, they found that a plant-powered diet brought some serious advantages: significantly lower rates of heart disease, stroke, cancer and type 2 diabetes. (24) People with the healthiest diets were 22% less likely to die from any cause during the 24 years that researchers followed them up!

Joining the plant-based diet revolution isn't about becoming 'vegan' or applying any other label to your diet or lifestyle. It's about simply choosing to build most of your meals (or all of them) from the foods that have consistently been shown to benefit human health. The weight of scientific evidence overwhelmingly favours a whole-food, plant-based diet as the optimal choice for human health and longevity. The more plant-based, the better.

THE THREE QUESTIONS I ASK EVERY PATIENT

Every medical student knows that the key to reaching an accurate diagnosis and treatment plan is to simply listen. One of the first things trainee doctors are taught is to pay careful attention to the details of each patient's story. This is called 'history taking' and it follows a particular sequence. We start by asking about the main problem or 'presenting complaint'. We then move on to more specific questions, asking when the problem started, if it has ever happened before and whether there is anything that makes it worse. Even more detailed questions about symptoms may then follow. Listening with great attention to each patient's story can be far more important than taking blood tests, requesting CT scans or even checking the patient's pulse. A doctor who has learned to listen well is far more likely to reach the correct diagnosis. (25)

Given the connection between food and health, I am constantly surprised to find that by the time patients come to my clinic, no one will have asked them to speak about the foods they eat every day. In a world of ten-minute appointments and busy waiting rooms, I can understand how many doctors might feel like they just don't have time to get into all that. We are all constantly working against the clock, but taking just a few minutes to ask every patient three simple questions about food can start a powerful conversation.

1. How many pieces of fruit do you eat each day?

2. How many servings of vegetables do you eat each day?

3. How many servings of wholegrains do you eat each day?

WHAT DO THREE SERVINGS OF FRUITS, VEGETABLES AND WHOLEGRAINS LOOK LIKE?

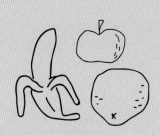

FRUITS

1 small apple +
1 large banana +
1 large orange

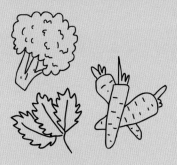

VEGETABLES

1 cereal bowl of leafy greens +
3 heaped tablespoons of any veg +
3 heaped tablespoons of beans

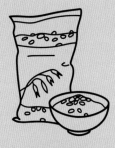

WHOLEGRAINS

3 tablespoons of cooked porridge +
1 slice of wholegrain bread +
3 tablespoons of cooked brown rice

These three simple questions are a great starting point for talking to my patients about the importance of a healthy approach to food. Are they reaching the modest 'five-a-day' recommendation for fruit and vegetable intake? Are they getting the recommended three servings of wholegrains per day? Are they eating any wholegrains at all? I'm hoping that they'll answer 'at least three' to each question. How did you do on these three questions? Do your numbers add up to nine or more? If not, we have identified your first target for healthy dietary change!

THE WHOLE-FOOD, PLANT-BASED APPROACH

Moving to a whole-food, plant-based diet means building your meals from fresh wholefoods that come from plants. These foods are consumed in unprocessed or minimally processed forms. By following this principle while eating to your natural appetite, your diet will be rich in the nutrients your body needs to thrive. (26-34) This has been consistently rated as one of most nutrient-rich dietary patterns available to humans, meaning that most of the common deficiencies that drive poor health are far less likely to occur. A healthy plant-based diet contains more fibre, folate, vitamins A, C and E, thiamine, riboflavin, magnesium, healthy oils, copper and iron than a diet that includes meat and dairy. (35-37)

WHAT ARE NUTRIENTS, ANYWAY?

Instead of describing the foods that we should eat, dietary guidelines often focus on individual nutrients, such as protein, carbohydrates, fats, oils, iron and calcium. These are the substances that the human body requires to function. In my opinion this is an artificial approach and doesn't really help people to make healthy food choices. Nonetheless, it's worth understanding what these terms refer to.

PROTEINS are used by the body to build muscles and connective tissues, such as tendons and cartilage. They are also used to make numerous hormones and enzymes, and are important for growth and repair. Your body makes proteins from building blocks called amino acids. Proteins make up about 15% of your body weight.

CARBOHYDRATES are the sugars and starches found in fruits, vegetables, grains and other plant-based foods. They are the body's main energy source and an important part of any healthy diet. Whole plant foods are a rich source of the complex carbohydrates that help our bodies to thrive. Various processing techniques are used to break down these complex carbohydrates and extract simple or refined sugars, such as glucose, sucrose and fructose, which are added to processed foods or sold as table sugar, syrups and sweeteners.

FATS AND OILS are energy-dense foods that are crucial to human health. Oils are simply fats that are liquid at room temperature. Our body uses fat as its main store of energy. We need dietary fats to produce hormones and to support the function of our brain and nervous system. They also provide essential fatty acids and fat-soluble vitamins. Certain types of dietary fats and oils are healthier than others. Fruits, vegetables, beans, nuts, seeds and wholegrains naturally contain healthy unsaturated plant-based oils in varying amounts. Meat and dairy on the other hand are rich sources of unhealthy saturated fats and cholesterol. (38-39)

VITAMINS AND MINERALS are substances that the body needs in small amounts to work properly and to stay healthy. For example, vitamin C is used for growth and repair in all parts of the body, while iron is essential for producing blood and transporting oxygen around your body. Iron is also needed to manufacture the genes that are found in almost every human cell.

ANTIOXIDANTS are substances that help the body to prevent or slow the damage that cells experience every day. Although the body can produce some antioxidants, we depend mostly on food to provide them. Vitamin C, beta-carotene, flavonoids, flavones, catechins, phenols and polyphenols are all types of antioxidant, and they are all found in plant-based foods.

PHYTONUTRIENTS are chemicals that occur naturally in plants ('phyto' comes from the Greek word for plant). Many of these chemicals are not needed to keep you alive, but consuming them can help to prevent disease and improve your health. All plant foods contain phytonutrients, but brightly coloured fruits and vegetables are especially good sources.

When it comes to fruits and vegetables, fewer than one in three adults make it to the modest five-a-day target.

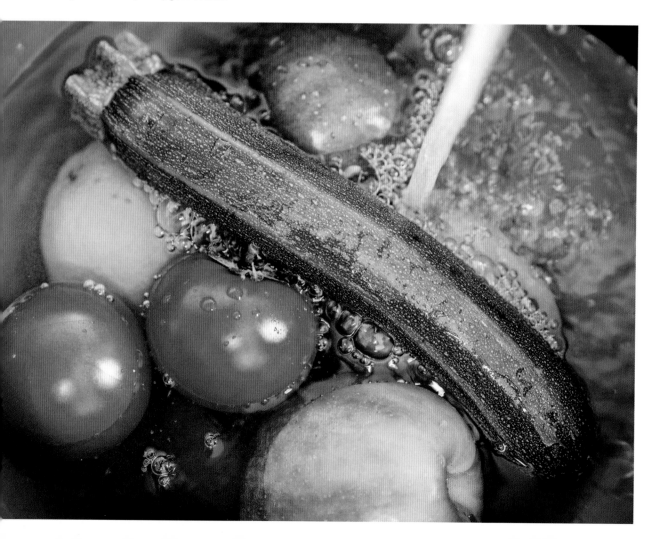

Wholegrains, beans, greens and legumes have been pushed out in favour of fast food, take-aways, processed meat pies and white bread bacon butties.

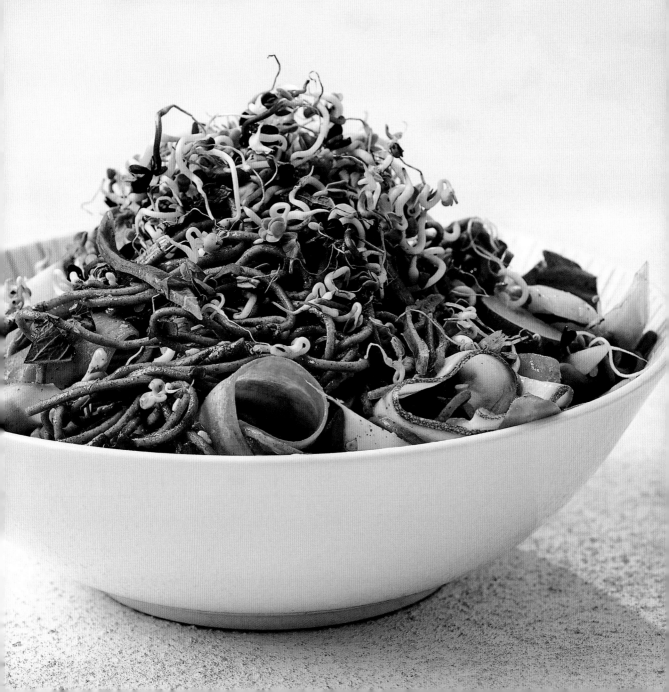

KEY NUTRIENTS ON A HEALTHY PLANT-BASED DIET

As you can see, a varied plant-based diet is naturally packed with important nutrients

HIGH-CALORIE FOODS
Porridge/oats
Sourdough bread
Medjool dates
Macadamia nuts
Roasted peanuts
Brown rice
Cashews
Pistachio nuts
White potato with skin
Avocado

PROTEIN
Legume pasta
Tofu/tempeh
Sourdough bread
Oats
Black beans
Lentils
Kidney beans
Peanuts (dry-roasted)
Chickpeas
Pistachio nuts

COMPLEX CARBOHYDRATES
Medjool dates
Sourdough bread
Oats
Potato, boiled with skin
Sweet potato
Brown rice
Mango
White rice
Quinoa
Pear

FAT
Macadamia nuts
Peanuts (dry roasted)
Avocado
Cashews
Pistachio nuts
Peanut butter
Brazil nuts
Pumpkin seeds
Flaxseeds
Chia seeds

POTASSIUM
White potato with skin
Sweet potato
Medjool dates
Avocado
Tomato
Mango
Black beans
Banana
Lentils
Pistachio nuts

MAGNESIUM
Cacao powder
Porridge/oats
Quinoa
Cashews
Potato (whole)
Brazil nuts
Pumpkin seeds
Brown rice
Chia seeds
Peanuts (dry roasted)

CALCIUM
Kale
Chia seeds
Sweet potato
Black beans
Collard greens
Medjool dates
Kidney beans
White potato
Oranges, raw
Calcium-set tofu
Fortified plant milks

IRON
White potato with skin
Sourdough bread
Lentils
Oats
Chia seeds
Black beans
Tofu
Quinoa
Cashews
Cacao powder

PHOSPHORUS
Porridge/oats
Quinoa
Lentils
Hemp seeds
Potato with skin
Cashews
Pistachio nuts
Brown rice
Black beans
Legumes

WATER
Fresh mango
Watermelon
Orange
Tomato
Soy milk
Apple
Pear
Sweet potato with skin
White potato with skin
Papaya

SELENIUM
Brazil nuts
Porridge/oats
Sourdough bread
Tofu
White rice
Brown rice
Chia seeds
Hemp seeds
Quinoa
Cashews (roasted)

OMEGA 3
Flaxseeds
Chia seeds
Black beans
Hemp seeds
Walnuts
Kale, raw
Quinoa
Mango
Avocado
Pecans

OMEGA 6
Pecans
Brazil nuts
Peanuts (dry roasted)
Peanut butter
Pistachio nuts
Pumpkin seeds
Tofu
Avocado
Cashews
Hemp seeds

ZINC
Porridge/oats
White potato with skin
Cashews
Quinoa
Cacao powder
Lentils
Tofu
Brown rice
Black beans
Pecans

VITAMIN K
Kale
Collard greens
Baby spinach
Brussels sprouts
Chia seeds
Broccoli
Kiwi fruit
Green peas
Rocket
Pistachio nuts

VITAMIN E
Sunflower seeds
Mango
Peanut butter
Avocado
Peanuts (dry roasted)
Red capsicum
Kiwi fruit
Sweet potato with skin
Brazil nuts
Tomato

VITAMIN C
Red capsicum
Kiwi fruit
Fresh mango
Papaya
Oranges
Broccoli
Pineapple
Brussels sprouts
Sweet potato with skin
Kale

VITAMIN A
Sweet potato with skin
Carrot
Red capsicum
Mango
Green peas
Spinach
Kale
Tomato
Collard greens
Papaya

B VITAMINS
Sweet potato
Sourdough
White potato with skin
Pistachio nuts
Avocado
Peanuts
Porridge/oats
Brown rice
Green peas
B12 supplement

CHOLINE
Black beans
White potato with skin
Tofu
Chickpeas
Green peas
Quinoa
Lentils
Porridge/oats
Kidney beans
Sweet potato

HOW TO EAT LIKE THE HEALTHIEST PEOPLE ON THE PLANET

You'll find all the recipes you need to start your revolution in Part 3. For now, let's examine the basic food groups that make up a healthy plant-based diet.

FRUITS AND VEGETABLES: The benefits gained from making these nutrient-packed foods a mainstay of your diet are truly astounding. According to researchers at University College London, people who eat seven or more portions a day are 31% less likely to die from heart disease. (40)

BEANS, NUTS AND SEEDS: Beans and other legumes or pulses (peas, lentils and chickpeas) are packed with the protein that your body needs to thrive, and are also rich in healthy oils, fibre, vitamins, minerals and antioxidants. Alongside nuts and seeds, they are great options for making you feel full, and also help to maintain a healthy body weight. Choosing to obtain your protein from these plant-based sources has multiple advantages, reducing your risk of obesity, heart disease, type 2 diabetes and numerous cancers. (41-50) Beans, nuts and seeds should make up about a quarter of your food.

WHOLEGRAINS: This group includes wheat, barley, brown rice, millet, oats, buckwheat and more besides. The healthiest populations in the world love these foods. Choosing wholegrains instead of processed or refined grains means that you are getting the benefits of the bran and germ layers of the grain, which are packed with fibre, protein and other important nutrients. Ensuring that a variety of wholegrains make up about a quarter of your food will help to add healthy years to your life. (51)

ADDED OILS: Fruits, vegetables, beans, nuts, seeds and wholegrains all naturally contain healthy plant-based oils in varying amounts. There is no real need to add extra oils to your food on a regular basis. You'll notice that our recipes sometimes include extra virgin olive oil as an option because its high content of mono-unsaturated fatty acids and phenols have been linked to reducing inflammation and helping to prevent heart disease. (52-55) If it helps you to enjoy your plant-based diet even more, by all means include it, but remember that oil contains a lot of calories. I recommend keeping it to roughly two tablespoons per day and regarding it as an optional extra.

SEASONING, HERBS AND SPICES: Black pepper, chilli flakes, cinnamon, ginger, turmeric, rosemary and more. Not only do herbs and spices add layers of flavour to your meals, they increase the diversity of plants on your plate, and come with powerful health benefits of their own. (56) The techniques you'll learn while preparing our recipes will ensure that you never again sit down to a bland plate of food.

DRINKS: When it comes to staying hydrated, the healthiest option is always a glass of clean drinking water. Plain old water with ice and a slice beats sweetened beverages every time. If you like tea or coffee, those are fine too.

ADDED SUGARS: Excess consumption of the simple refined sugars found in sweets and processed foods is a major driver of poor health. Our recipes occasionally use maple syrup, which counts as an added sugar, but we keep the amount low. Try to keep your use of all refined and added sugars to a minimum. Super-sweet foods should be a rare and occasional treat.

Ensuring that a variety of wholegrains make up about a quarter of your food will help to add healthy years to your life.

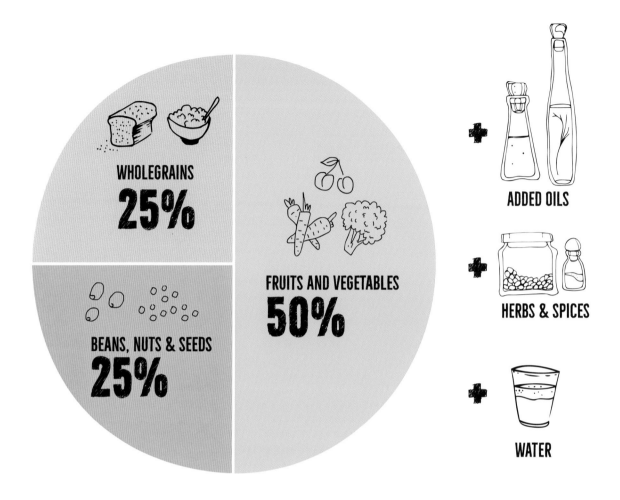

The plant-based diet revolution has already started! Recent figures indicate that two-thirds of people are actively reducing their intake of meat, and a quarter of new food products launched in the UK are completely plant-based. As a doctor, I couldn't be happier. As members of the public of all ages turn to eating more plants, we can look forward to seeing less chronic disease. The future looks brighter. But don't take it from me – take it from the world's largest professional body for dietitians, the American Academy of Nutrition and Dietetics:

It is the position of the Academy of Nutrition and Dietetics that appropriately planned vegetarian, including vegan, diets are healthful, nutritionally adequate, and may provide health benefits for the prevention and treatment of certain diseases. These diets are appropriate for all stages of the life cycle, including pregnancy, lactation, infancy, childhood, adolescence, older adulthood, and for athletes. Vegetarians and vegans are at reduced risk of certain health conditions, including ischaemic heart disease, type 2 diabetes, hypertension, certain types of cancer, and obesity. (57)

Whatever your age and whatever your stage of life, a whole-food, plant-based diet is a great option.

PLANT-BASED OR MEDITERRANEAN?

Many doctors and dietitians correctly highlight the benefits of the traditional diet found in Mediterranean countries such as France, Greece, Italy and Spain. This poses a big question: does embracing a whole-food, plant-based diet mean missing out on the benefits of a Mediterranean diet? High in vegetables, fruit, nuts, seeds, legumes and olive oil, the classically described Mediterranean diet originated in peasant communities, where people had limited access to meat and dairy products. Far from being deprived, those communities tended to be extremely healthy.

Dietitians and researchers have developed numerous scoring systems to rate an individual's diet according to 'how Mediterranean' they are eating. In a study published by the *International Journal of Food Sciences and Nutrition*, (58) researchers applied one such scoring system to the diets of 1,230 healthy volunteers, a mix of vegans, vegetarians and meat-eaters.

They found that those eating a completely plant-based diet were 32 times more likely than meat-eaters to reach or exceed the standard for an extremely healthy 'Mediterranean diet'. Those eating a vegetarian diet (with dairy and eggs) were just three times more likely to make the grade. This doesn't surprise me. A whole-food, plant-based diet is built from the healthiest components of the classic Mediterranean diet: legumes, wholegrains, fruits, vegetables, nuts and seeds. As you tuck into a plate of Farinata with courgettes, tomatoes & capers (see page 92), you might wonder 'Is this dish Mediterranean or vegan?' It turns out that a whole-food, plant-based meal is the healthiest version of both!

> Those eating a completely plant-based diet were 32 times more likely than meat-eaters to reach or exceed the standard for an extremely healthy Mediterranean diet.

THE SIX SUPERFOODS THAT REDUCE YOUR RISK OF DISEASE AND PROTECT THE PLANET

In the 21st century, 40% of global deaths are caused by diseases strongly linked to poor-quality diet, and the environment is struggling under the pressures of food production. Top researchers from the Universities of Oxford, Minnesota and California recently joined forces to figure out what we can do about it. (59) Combining the results from dozens of studies, they examined the links between 15 food groups and 34 health outcomes, focusing on type 2 diabetes, stroke, heart disease, bowel cancer and life expectancy. They correlated their results with the known environmental impact of producing the same 15 food groups. The super six were:

- WHOLEGRAINS
- FRUITS
- VEGETABLES
- LEGUMES
- NUTS
- OLIVE OIL

These foods consistently reduce the risk of multiple disease outcomes and increase longevity. In other words, they make for a healthier and longer life. They also have the lowest impact on the environment and planetary health.

Red meat and processed meats came out as the super-villains of this story, simultaneously increasing the risk of multiple diseases and shortening life expectancy, while having the maximum impact on water use, land use and greenhouse gas emissions. In fact, every animal product studied failed to make the superfood category. The reasons I recommend a whole-food, plant-based diet are firmly rooted in the medical evidence. But I'm keenly aware that a global scientific consensus agrees that by filling our plates with foods of plant origin we are also doing Mother Nature a big favour.

SHOULD I BUY ORGANIC?

Organic fruits and vegetables are produced without using artificial chemical pesticides, and sometimes have the benefit of containing higher levels of antioxidants and many other nutrients. Organic fruits and veg also come with far lower amounts of chemical pesticide residue. This may be important, as some of these chemicals can accumulate in the body over time. Buying organic can be more expensive, so is not available to everyone. My advice is to buy the best-quality produce available within your budget. Buying organic should not be viewed as an essential part of your move to a healthier diet. Certain fruits and vegetables come with minimal pesticide residue even if they've been produced by conventional, non-organic means. (60)

The following produce come with very little pesticide residue even if you don't buy organic: avocados, asparagus, aubergine, broccoli, cabbage, cantaloupe melon, cauliflower, frozen peas, honeydew melon, kiwi fruit, mushrooms, onions, papaya, pineapple and sweetcorn.

Conventional growing of the following produce can require significant use of pesticides, so it may be worth buying these from the organic section, if possible: apples, celery, cherries, grapes, kale, nectarines, peaches, pears, potatoes, spinach, strawberries and tomatoes.

Whether you buy organic or conventional, always wash your fruit and veg before eating.

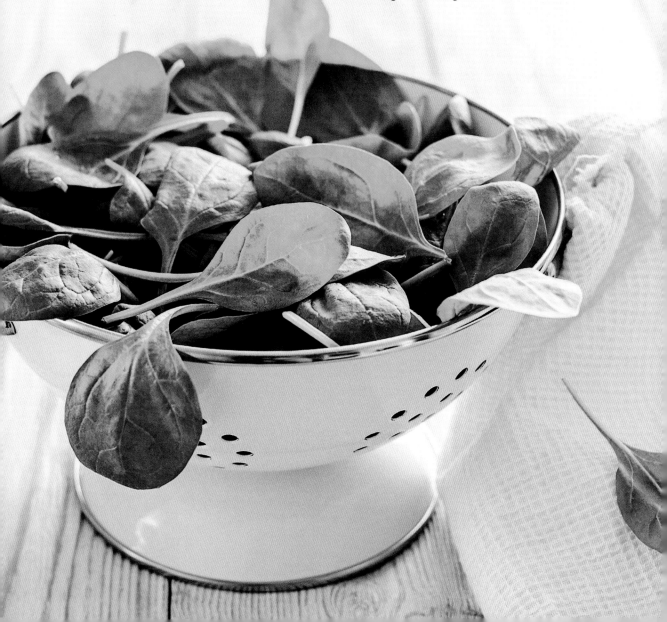

DOCTOR'S ORDERS:
TEN PRESCRIPTIONS FOR BETTER HEALTH

Evidence-based dietary advice has become an incredibly important part of my medical practice. In a country where poor diet causes more illnesses than alcohol and drug abuse combined, (61) it could be argued that food should be a mandatory part of the conversation every time you meet a doctor. Here are the ten food-focused prescriptions I wish I could give to every person seeking to improve their health.

PRESCRIPTION 1

EAT A DIVERSITY OF PLANTS

The key to a healthy plant-based diet is variety. Learning to prepare and cook a wide range of vegetables, fruits, wholegrains and legumes will be an essential part of your journey. In the past you might have depended on a narrow range of plants to fill the veg section on your plate. Bestsellers, such as broccoli, courgettes, cucumbers and potatoes, are fantastic, but to increase the variety of plants on your plate you'll need to broaden your choices. You'll be delighted by the complex and delicious flavours waiting to be discovered in humble plants like aubergines, cabbages and chickpeas.

By maximising the number of different plants in your diet, you'll reap the benefits of a wider range of plant-derived nutrients, antioxidants, complex carbohydrates, proteins and beneficial fats. As you'll learn later, the all-important microbes of your gut microbiome thrive when you maximise the diversity of plants in your diet.

PRESCRIPTION 2

DITCH THE JUNK

The food industry uses the term 'ultra-processed food' to describe items like mass-produced cakes and pastries, packaged chips and crisps, soft drinks, chocolate, instant noodles and processed meat products, such as chicken nuggets and meatballs. The more common term for these products is 'junk food'. In 2018 a large study showed that UK adults get more than half their calories from junk foods, and only one-third of calories from foods in their natural state. Alarmingly, one in five of those surveyed were getting a massive 80% of their calories from ultra-processed foods. (62)

Depending on these products means missing out on the benefits of wholefoods, while increasing your intake of added sugars, unhealthy fats and sodium. Add to this the artificial flavours, sweeteners and emulsifiers that we know are bad news for our health and its clear why this junk food obsession is causing so much harm. In later chapters you'll learn more about the damage ultra-processed foods can cause and why they pose such a threat to the most important allies you have on your journey to better health – the trillions of micro-organisms that make up your gut microbiome.

PRESCRIPTION 3

EAT WHOLEGRAINS EVERY DAY

Eating wholegrains increases your chances of a long and healthy life. To quote from one major scientific review of the evidence: 'Wholegrain intake is associated with reduced risk of coronary heart disease, cardiovascular disease, and total cancer, and mortality from all causes, respiratory diseases, infectious diseases, diabetes, and all non-cardiovascular, non-cancer causes.' (63) And it's not just about wholegrain bread and high-fibre breakfast cereals! I want you to explore everything the wholegrain world has to offer. Barley, brown rice, millet, oats, freekeh and buckwheat are all great options. Did you know that popcorn is a wholegrain? Breakfast is a great time to start your daily wholegrain intake, so check out the perfect porridge and easy bread recipes on pages 64 and 70.

PRESCRIPTION 4

EMBRACE WHOLE CARBOHYDRATES

The plant-based diet revolution does not involve avoiding all carbohydrates. In fact, it's the opposite of a low-carb diet. By eating plenty of whole carbohydrates, you are giving your body the fibre, fuel and nutrients it needs. Cutting out healthy carbohydrates means depriving yourself of some of the most beneficial foods known to nutritional science. Trying to combine 'whole-food, plant-based' with 'low-carb' is one of the commonest mistakes I have seen in people making the switch to plants. Oats, rice, wholegrains, bananas, strawberries, apples and potatoes (all sources of carbohydrate) are incredibly beneficial foods. Indeed, avoiding them can leave you feeling hungry and lethargic. In the long term, low-carb diets can put you at risk of multiple health problems, so healthy whole carbohydrates are definitely on the plant-based menu. As you embark on the 28-Day Revolution meal plans (see page 200), you'll be getting approximately 60% of your calories from whole carbohydrates. The science shows that making these healthy carbohydrates part of your daily diet improves your health and adds good years to your life. (63-68)

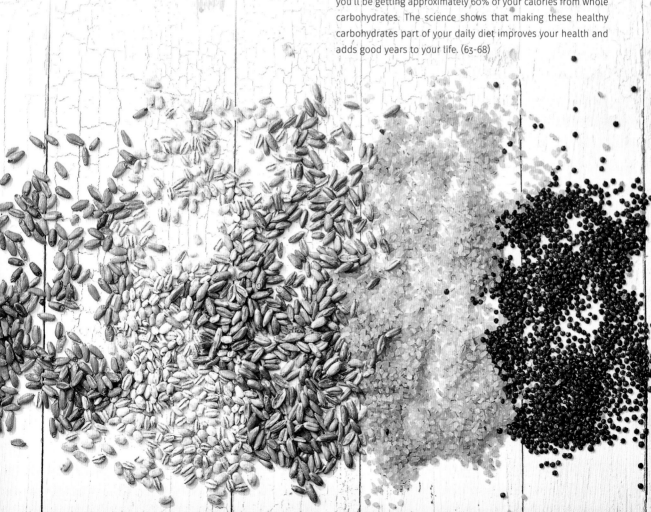

PRESCRIPTION 5

CHOOSE YOUR PROTEIN WISELY

One of the most enduring myths about a plant-based diet is that it leads to protein deficiency. It's just not true. Here's the secret: all plants contain protein! Look at some of the recipes in Part 3 right now. You'll be surprised by just how much protein these plant-based dishes pack in. Summer veg & white bean pasta: 35g per portion. Rosti pie with braised cabbage & peas: 24g per portion. Even two slices of our Brown soda bread provides you with an impressive 26g of plant-based protein.

The average adult requires about 42g of protein per day. In 2014 researchers analysed the dietary intake of 71,000 US and Canadian adults. (69) The group included 33,600 non-vegetarians and 5,700 strict vegetarians who ate animal products less than once per month. The results showed that both groups were getting about 70g of protein per day. While choosing plants over meat, 95% of strict vegetarians were exceeding their daily protein needs. In fact, the top 5% were getting close to 100g of protein per day.

Thanks to the fact that all plants contain protein, the 28-Day Revolution meal plans (see page 200) provide about 70g of healthy plant-based protein each day, more than enough for the average active person. If you need more protein, simply eat more food!

Choosing to get your protein from plants instead of from meat and other animal products may be one of the healthiest decisions you can make, reducing your risk of inflammatory bowel disease, heart disease, bowel cancer, type 2 diabetes, and many other chronic diseases. You'll even avoid causing harmful changes in your gut microbiome. (70-86)

PRESCRIPTION 6

TAKE A VITAMIN B12 SUPPLEMENT

Vitamin B12 is an important part of the human diet, essential for normal red blood cell formation, neurological function and DNA synthesis. Without enough vitamin B12 you are at risk of developing anaemia, extreme fatigue, poor mental functioning, tingling and numbness in your limbs, and poor overall health. (87)

Vitamin B12 is made by certain soil bacteria. Ancient humans were never clean. The plants they ate were covered with soil and acted as sources of vitamin B12. Back then it was even in the drinking water. (88) Because our fruits and vegetables are now washed and cleaned of any soil prior to eating, they no longer come with a source of vitamin B12. Deficiency is common, no matter what sort of diet you eat. (89) I don't recommend eating soil, but I do strongly recommend taking a vitamin B12 supplement.

Older studies showed that vitamin B12 deficiency occurs in all dietary patterns but is more likely in vegetarians. (91) In recent years, this trend has started to reverse. Health-conscious vegetarians and vegans are now less likely than meat-eaters to have vitamin B12 deficiency. (90-91) Why? Because they've read the science and have started to supplement. In my view, taking a vitamin B12 supplement is a mandatory part of maintaining a healthy plant-based diet.

The body needs just 2.4 micrograms (mcg) per day, but you need to take more than this because it's not fully absorbed. To keep things simple, I recommend a supplement called VEG-1. It contains 25mcg of highly absorbable vitamin B12 (called cyanocobalamin) and your daily doses of vitamin D, as well as iodine and selenium, which are hard to plan for on any diet. It costs just £25 for a one-year supply and profits go to charity. You can order VEG-1 for worldwide delivery at www.vegansociety.com. There are hundreds of other great brands available. The body's ability to absorb vitamin B12 decreases with age. If you are over 65, or have a history of deficiency, doses of up to 1000mcg once a day can be safely recommended. (92)

PRESCRIPTION 7

CUT DOWN ON THE SWEET STUFF

Our primitive brains may be programmed to enjoy sweeter foods, but there's no getting away from the fact that purified sugar is not a healthy choice. Despite national guidelines that added sugars should not exceed 5% of our total energy intake, adults are currently eating over twice this much, averaging 50–60g (12–15 teaspoons) of added sugar per day. (93)

Luckily for us, the natural sugars contained in whole fruits and vegetables do not have these effects and are not regarded as added sugars. The major sources of added sugars are sugary drinks, sweets and pastries. I strongly advise you to keep those foods and drinks out of reach as you embark on your own health revolution. Some of our recipes do include a little added sugar in the form of maple syrup, but feel free to use less, or even none at all.

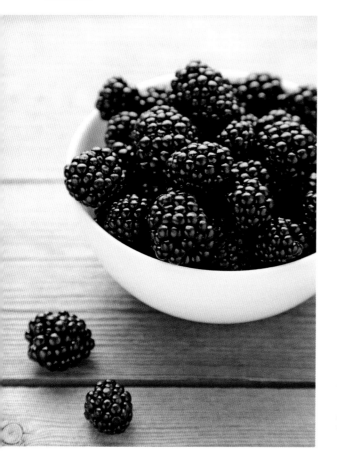

PRESCRIPTION 8

REMEMBER THAT MILK IS FOR BABIES!

Milk, cheese and yogurt have long been promoted as good sources of calcium, and beneficial and even necessary for human health. While human breast milk is the perfect food for a baby, and cow's milk is the perfect food for a calf, for adult humans the benefits of regular milk consumption are not so evident. In 2020, the *New England Journal of Medicine* published a review of the evidence on milk and health. (94) The conclusions were clear: the health claims often used by the dairy industry do not stand up. Indeed, consuming dairy foods may increase your risk of bone fractures, heart disease and various common cancers.

When it comes to getting the calcium your body needs, plant-based sources, such as broccoli, tofu, nuts and beans, are far healthier options. When you add to this science the fact that up to three-quarters of adults lack the enzyme required to digest dairy foods, leading to bloating and distressing abdominal symptoms, I have no hesitation in recommending a dairy-free diet. (95)

The 28-Day Revolution meal plans (see page 200) are packed with plant-based sources of calcium and provide an average of 780mg per day. This is well over the recommended daily intake for a healthy adult. If your doctor has advised you to consume more calcium than this, you can top up by eating more of the healthy calcium-rich foods listed on page 17.

When it comes to getting the calcium your body needs, plant-based sources, such as broccoli, tofu, nuts and beans, are far healthier options.

PRESCRIPTION 9

DON'T FORGET YOUR SUNSHINE VITAMIN

Whether your diet is completely plant-based, flexitarian or omnivore, you are at risk of vitamin D deficiency, which has been linked to increased risk of fracture, cognitive impairment, poor dental health, reduced muscle strength, falls in the elderly, cancer risk, poor outcomes in inflammatory bowel disease, heart disease, high blood pressure and a generally increased risk of dying. Active vitamin D is manufactured in the skin, but this process depends on exposure to sunlight. With 40 minutes of bright sunshine a day (20 minutes if you have lighter skin), your body can make all the vitamin D you need.

In a world where we tend to keep our skin covered up, spend our days indoors and live further from the Equator than our ancestors, vitamin D deficiency has become a real public health concern. The UK Scientific Advisory Committee on Nutrition recommends that everyone should take a vitamin D supplement during the winter months, or year-round if they work indoors. (96)

While you can obtain small amounts of vitamin D from foods such as tofu and mushrooms, and from fortified plant-based milks, if you cannot guarantee exposure to sufficient bright sunshine every day of the year, the best advice is to take 400–1000iu (10–25mcg) of vitamin D each day. (96) The VEG-1 multivitamin mentioned earlier contains adequate vitamin D alongside your daily dose of vitamin B12 and other important trace nutrients, such as iodine and selenium, which are difficult to plan for on any diet. Higher doses of vitamin D can be harmful, so only take doses greater than 2000iu (50mcg) daily if recommended by your doctor.

PRESCRIPTION 10

GET HELP IF YOU NEED IT

In Part 2, Unlocking the Plant-based Advantage, you'll discover the science showing exactly how a plant-based diet can substantially reduce your risk of illness and help to treat many chronic diseases. I've seen this science played out in my clinic and will share several of my patients' success stories with you. However, there is no dietary change that can make a person disease-proof! If you have ongoing symptoms or suspect that you have an underlying health problem, it's always a good idea to talk to your family doctor, specialist or practice nurse. If you are making the switch to plants to manage high blood pressure, high cholesterol or any health issue, please keep your medical team updated so that they can support you in this healthy change. If you experience new symptoms while making the switch to a plant-based diet, particularly if you have a pre-existing gut health issue, such as a genuine food intolerance or inflammatory bowel disease, the assistance of a registered dietitian can be invaluable. Seeking help is not a failure, it's just the smart thing to do.

With 40 minutes of bright sunshine a day (20 minutes if you have lighter skin), your body can make all the vitamin D you need.

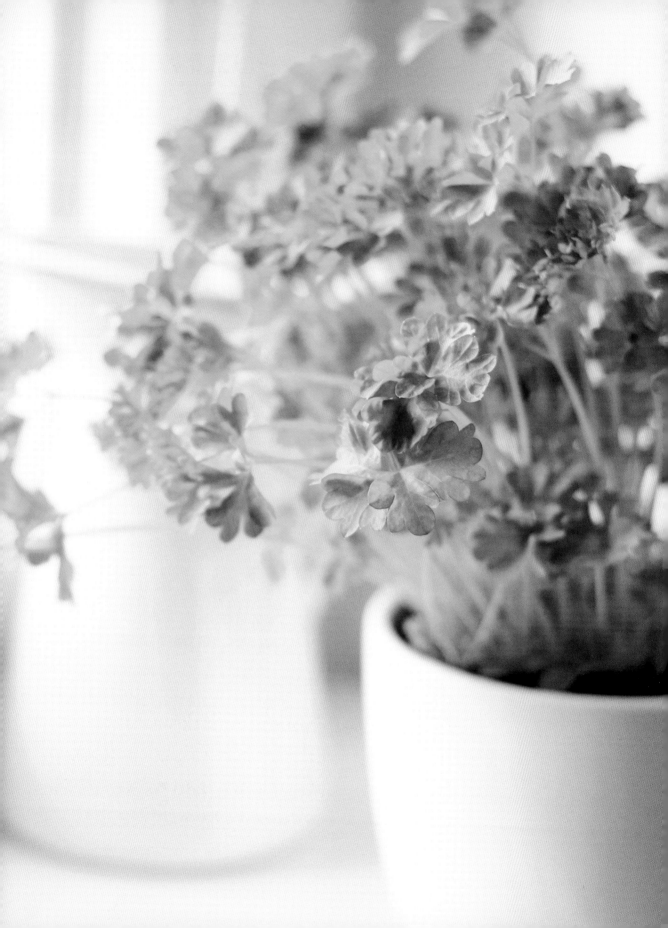

PART TWO

UNLOCKING THE PLANT-BASED ADVANTAGE

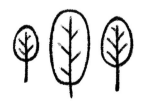

HEALTHY GUT

———

We are not alone. There are more micro-organisms living within each of our digestive systems than there are trees on planet Earth or stars in the Milky Way. (97-99) Each one of us carries about 100 trillion microbes in our gut. These microscopic bacteria, archae, viruses and yeasts make up your gut microbiome, which contains ten times more cells and 100 times more genetic material than the rest of your body combined. As you embark on your plant-based diet revolution, the friendly microbes of your gut microbiome will become your crucial allies.

The human microbiome consists of a vast diversity of microscopic organisms with wonderful names like *Clostridiales* bacterium and *Bilophila wadsworthia*. They are the descendants of the earth's first living inhabitants, clusters of single-celled organisms that emerged between two and four billion years ago. They have been with humans on every step of our evolutionary journey. Our personal microbiome begins to form at birth. With our first breath and our first human touch, our microbial population begins to take shape. (100) Our new microbes get to work quickly, helping us to digest our very first meal. Our mother's milk doesn't just provide calories, it also contains live beneficial bacteria (probiotics) and substances to promote the growth of our own healthy bacteria (prebiotics). This early process of 'seeding' helps to define our developing microbiome and may be the mechanism by which breastfeeding protects children from certain illnesses, including asthma and type 1 diabetes. (101)

Our microbes are also crucial in helping our new-born gut to develop. They promote the growth of its delicate blood supply, provide important enzymes, and help to ensure that the lining of the gut develops correctly. Our microbes also produce specific proteins to ward off potentially harmful bacteria and other infections. Without our gut bacteria, the critically important immune system of the gut would not develop or function effectively. (102) By the time we reach the age of two, our gut microbiome has taken on its mature form. Although your personal collection of gut bugs is unique and completely individual to you, it remains remarkably adaptable. Throughout your adult life your gut microbiome continues to respond to your gut environment and the foods that you eat. Although we have been aware of the lowly bugs living in our gut since 1681 (these tiny living organisms were initially described as 'animalcules'!), the pivotal role that they play in our health and well-being has really only emerged in the last twenty years. The human gut microbiome is now recognised as a 'control centre for human biology'. (104-5)

YOUR GUT MICROBIOME LOVES FIBRE

The human body can't digest fibre, but our healthy microbes thrive on it. (104) The term 'fibre' refers to dozens of structural carbohydrates that are found only in plants. These complex carbohydrates are essential to maintain a health-promoting gut microbiome. When you have porridge oats for breakfast or wholegrain bread with lunch, your gut microbes soon get to work breaking down the fibre through the process of 'fermentation'. This process provides our healthy bugs with the energy they need to thrive. The more plant fibres you feed those beneficial bugs, the more they grow and replicate. The result of fermentation is a steady supply of the most beneficial products that you've never heard of: short-chain fatty acids (SCFAs). Within days of switching to a high-fibre diet, the number of fibre-loving bacteria in your personal gut microbiome will begin to surge. (105) And more fibre-loving bugs means more SCFAs!

Those SCFAs have so many benefits to our health that it's hard to keep up with the research. For example, they bind directly to specialised cells in the gut lining, turning on the production of hormones called GLP-1 and Peptide YY. These hormones signal to the body that we've had enough to eat so that we don't consume too many calories. They also help to control blood sugar levels, which is critically important for the healthy functioning of our brain and other essential organs. SCFAs act as an energy source for the cells that line the large bowel and directly activate the immune cells in the gut lining, encouraging them to maintain an effective gut barrier. Without a steady supply of fibre and the resulting SCFAs, the gut lining quickly becomes unhealthy and more permeable. A fibre-starved gut can become a 'leaky gut' – one that allows harmful bacterial products and toxins to enter the bloodstream. (106-7)

To the outside observer it seems like our fibre-loving microbes produce SCFAs with the clear goal of keeping their human host as healthy as possible for as long as possible. It should come as no surprise to you that people who eat less fibre produce much lower levels of these incredibly beneficial chemicals. (108) Fibre deficiency is just one of the ways that the Standard Western Diet damages our gut microbial health. As you'll learn in later chapters, the constant supply of saturated fats, added sugars, meat and refined grains that come with the modern diet all combine to promote a microbiome that is enriched with harmful bacteria. This dysfunctional version of a human gut microbiome sets us up for heart disease, obesity, type 2 diabetes and overall poor health. (109-10)

PLANT DIVERSITY IS KING!

Between 2012 and 2017 a team of US-based researchers set out to discover the factors that influence the health of the human gut microbiome in the industrialised world. (111) They completed a detailed analysis of more than 11,000 volunteers, most of whom lived in the UK, the USA and Australia. The results of what became known as the American Gut Project reveal that when it comes to food, the number one predictor of a healthy gut microbiome is the diversity of plants in your diet. Participants who ate more than 30 different plants per week had unique fibre-loving bacteria that just weren't found in people on a plant-deprived diet.

In the 21st century our global food supply depends on just 120 of the more than 250,000 different plants that humans could grow and eat. Varieties of just three plants (corn, wheat and rice) account for more than half of all food calories consumed in the world. (112) This means that our modern gut microbiomes never get to ferment 99.9% of the edible plants available on our planet! Among the 11,000 volunteers who took part in the American Gut Project, fewer than 1 in 250 were hitting that magic number of 30 different plants per week.

I'm not asking you to eat thousands of different fruits, vegetables, legumes and wholegrains, but I am strongly suggesting that we can all benefit from increasing the diversity of plants in our diets. Try it for a week. Keep a running total for each meal and snack to find out how many plants your microbes are getting to ferment. As you try out the recipes in this book, add their plant score to your total weekly number. Can you reach more than 30?

The 28-Day Revolution meal plans will truly max out your plant diversity, putting between 50 and 70 different plants on your plate each week. Your gut microbes are in for a treat!

HOW THE GUT MICROBIOME SAVED THE HUMAN RACE

The foods we eat are the major factor in deciding which of our microbes survive and thrive. Although each human microbiome is unique, every one falls into one of two broad groups or enterotypes. People who favour animal fat and meat tend to have a microbiome dominated by Bacteroides bacteria. Those who favour plants and eat lots of fibre have predominantly Prevotella bacteria. (113) Nowadays, most people eat pretty much the same foods whatever the season. Thanks to limited and repetitive diets, the adult human microbiome can go for years without significant variation in its make-up or metabolic functions. (114)

The gut microbiome of one of our closest living relatives is strikingly different. Western lowland gorillas share 98% of their genetic code with modern humans. Having split off from our evolutionary tree about 10 million years ago, they still live in their natural environment and eat a varied whole-food, plant-based diet, with no animal products (apart from the occasional termite). They spend most of their day foraging for edible plants. In stark contrast to modern humans, they consume over 200 species and varieties of plants and 100 species of fruits. Obtaining almost three quarters of their energy intake from such a rich diversity of plants means that our gorilla cousins are true super-fermenters. (115)

During periods of high-fruit availability, up to 70% of their feeding time is devoted to eating succulent fruits. As fruit becomes scarce, they shift to eating high volumes of various leaves, bark, herbs and fibrous fruits. (116) This ability to eat a radically different diet with the changing seasons is thanks to the rapid adaptation of the gut microbiome, which changes its structure and ability to digest different foods almost on demand. The flexibility of the gorilla microbiome gives a fascinating insight into how gut microbes benefited human survival in prehistoric times. When the environment and food availability shifted too rapidly for the human metabolism to adjust, gut microbes came to the rescue, quickly adapting to ensure that we could digest our food and absorb the nutrients we needed to survive and continue as a species. Thanks to our incredibly adaptable gut microbes, primitive humans were probably saved from extinction on many occasions.

There is a common microbiome thread linking us to our primate cousins even in the 21st century. The Prevotella enterotype still occurs in wild gorillas, chimpanzees and in present-day humans who eat a varied plant-based diet. This primitive and beneficial enterotype has largely died out in humans thanks to the Standard Western Diet, which is high in meat and dairy, high in artificial additives and low in plant diversity whatever the season. (117-18) For modern humans, a plant-based diet builds a gut microbiome with tremendous potential to improve health and well-being. The plant-powered microbiome is better at finding and breaking down nutrients, better at manufacturing essential amino acids, vitamins, SCFAs and other substances that make us healthier. (119) New papers on the microbiome advantages of eating plants are published almost daily. These studies encompass obesity, type 2 diabetes, heart disease, rheumatoid arthritis and even some early work in patients with Parkinson's disease. (120-21) Researchers have even tried giving patients a 'healthy vegan microbiome transplant' (also known as a 'vegan poop transplant') as a treatment for obesity, high cholesterol and insulin resistance! (122) You won't be surprised to learn that it worked, but only for a few days. Why? Because the researchers allowed the volunteers to continue eating the same Standard Western Diet that had made them unwell in the first place!

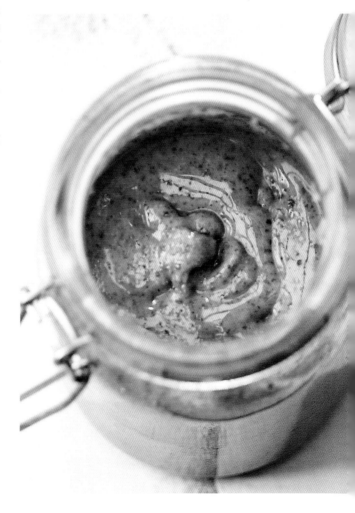

HOW JUNK FOODS ATTACK OUR GUT

Since the 1950s the food industry has used artificial fillers, flavour enhancers, emulsifiers and stabilisers to keep industrially produced foods fresh on the shelf and to make them taste like something you'd want to eat. Chemicals like maltodextrin, polysorbate-80 and carboxymethylcellulose are now manufactured in chemical factories and pumped into our food chain every day. Junk-food options like biscuits, mass-produced buns and breads, sweetened cereals, margarines and spreads, packaged snacks, ice cream, flavoured yogurts, fizzy drinks, powdered meals, ready-made meals, and instant sauces make up over half of all the calories we eat. (130, 131) These products truly are 'junk', not food. They have no business being in the human digestive system. Many of the industrial chemicals that they contain can attack our gut health.

Stretched out, the thin lining of our gut would cover an area about the size of a large garden. This large surface is needed to allow our gut to digest our food and to absorb the nutrients we need. Constantly exposed to bacteria, viruses, yeasts, toxins and the by-products of the foods we eat, the gut lining also provides a protective barrier between our gut contents and our bloodstream. Its job is to keep potentially harmful bugs and other substances from gaining access to our body. For much of its length this crucial barrier is made up of a single layer of cells covered by a thin coating of protective mucin. The junk-food chemicals that many of us eat two or three times a day launch a two-pronged attack on this line of defence: they promote the growth of harmful gut bacteria and actively degrade the barrier. Just like fibre-deficiency, this leads to a condition referred to as 'leaky gut', which allows harmful bacteria and their by-products to breach our defences, come in direct contact with our immune system and trigger abnormal inflammatory responses in our gut and beyond. (132-136)

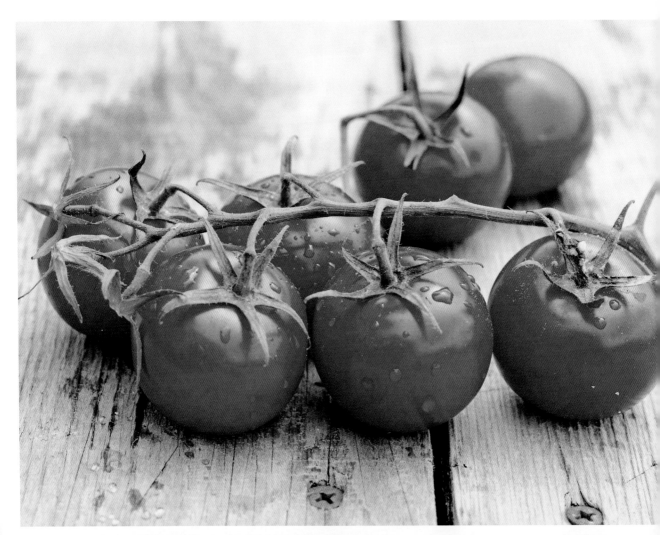

A TRULY ANTI-INFLAMMATORY DIET

Inflammation is an important process and one that is crucial to understand on your journey to better health. When faced with a threat such as a physical injury, infection, toxins and even the formation of early cancer cells, your body responds by increasing blood flow to the affected area, releasing specialised chemicals and increasing the numbers of immune cells present to tackle the threat. This short-term inflammatory response is essential to human health, designed to eliminate toxic agents and start the repair of damaged tissue. Once the threat has been dealt with, those inflammatory mechanisms are no longer needed and should switch off. If they remain active, your body enters a state referred to as 'chronic' inflammation, the long-term presence of a low-grade inflammatory response. This is an abnormal and unhealthy state. Chronic inflammation is a common factor linking Crohn's disease, obesity, type 2 diabetes, heart disease, stroke, arthritis, depression and many more disease states. (137)

The foods we choose to eat play a tremendous role in promoting or reducing chronic inflammation. Higher consumption of animal fat and animal protein has been shown to promote inflammation both in the gut and throughout the body. (138-146) The effect that these foods exert on our gut microbiome was illustrated in 2014 when a team of Harvard and University of California microbiome researchers asked ten healthy volunteers to eat a menu with lots of eggs, red meat, bacon and cheese for four days. Within 24 hours of adopting this 'animal-based diet' their pro-inflammatory bacteria flourished. (147)

The evidence favouring a more plant-based approach for combating chronic inflammation is compelling. Getting your calories from plants maximises your intake of anti-inflammatory compounds and antioxidants including flavonoids and carotenoids, vitamin C and vitamin E. A plant-based diet is also naturally higher in the healthy unsaturated fats that come from plants and is lower in the pro-inflammatory saturated fats and haem iron that come from animal products. (148-151) It's no surprise that multiple markers of chronic inflammation are lower in long-term vegans. Almost by definition, a plant-based diet truly is an 'anti-inflammatory diet'. This is one of the key benefits of taking a plant-based approach to the food on your plate.

By the time I'd qualified as a consultant gastroenterologist in 2012 my approach to treating severe gut inflammation had changed. As well as using the best medications available, I was ready to provide evidence-based answers to my patients' questions about food. I was actively educating my patients on how to move towards a 'whole-food, plant-based diet'. When it

FIBRE AND CROHN'S DISEASE

Patients with Crohn's disease, or the closely related condition ulcerative colitis, are often advised to adopt a very low-fibre diet. The logic has always been that less fibre means fewer bowel movements, which may help patients to manage their symptoms. However, that approach is not evidence-based and often does not lead to better outcomes. (167-168) Many of my patients have benefited greatly from moving to a predominantly or completely plant-based diet. Those with early and less severe disease have made the change by simply buying some good cookbooks and introducing more plant-based options over time. Others, especially those who have had surgery on the bowel, who have very active disease or narrowed segments of bowel due to inflammation, have benefited greatly from the individual support of my registered dietitian colleagues.

If you've been trying to manage the symptoms of Crohn's disease or ulcerative colitis with a very low-fibre diet, please talk to your dietitian. They can advise you how to make gradual increases in fibre. In one study, patients on a traditional low-fibre diet with mildly active Crohn's disease tolerated a modest increase in fibre – 12g per day – just fine, with all participants reporting reduced symptoms. (169) Many of the breakfasts, lighter meals and sweet treats in this book contain less than 12g of fibre per serving. Continue to work with your medical team. Healthy dietary changes and medications are equally important. When we are aiming for full health, we need to use every tool at our disposal!

came to treating Crohn's disease, meals that dramatically reduce or eliminate processed foods, dairy, animal fat and animal protein, while putting emphasis on plant-based sources of nutrition, put my patients in the best possible position to reverse gut inflammation, improve their symptoms, reduce disease activity and enter remission. (152-166) As I began to see results at my clinic, it was obvious that the benefits of a whole-food, plant-based diet went far beyond a healthier gut.

PLANT-BASED SUCCESS: JOHN'S STORY

John was a 72-year-old ex-military man, overweight and living with pre-diabetes. He'd been diagnosed with Crohn's disease of the large bowel several years previously and was doing okay on a low dose of immune-suppressing medication. When he first attended my clinic, his symptoms were manageable but still impacting on his quality of life. Like so many people with a chronic disease, John had simply learned to live with poor health. We reviewed his progress and talked about food. John loved barbecued steak and was eating a meat-heavy version of the standard British diet. On the surface he didn't immediately strike me as the ideal candidate for a plant-based overhaul, but we agreed on a few achievable goals: extra focus on beans, greens and wholegrains; no processed meat and no red meat at all. John even agreed to keep poultry to once or twice a week. I was impressed by his readiness for change.

Six months later, John sat in my office on a sunny July afternoon and all he wanted to talk about was food! He'd dropped 19kg (42lb) in excess weight and was no longer classed as obese. His blood sugar control had improved to the point that he no longer had pre-diabetes. He was truly thriving. We spent our 20-minute appointment exchanging the names of plant-based cookbooks and talking about his decision to throw away his barbecue. As he rose to leave, I asked one last question: 'We haven't really talked about your Crohn's disease today, John. Are you sure it's all right?' 'Absolutely, Doc. Never been better. We can talk about it the next time.' Patient visits like this started to become commonplace.

As I began to see results at my clinic, it became obvious that the benefits of a whole-food, plant-based diet went far beyond a healthier gut.

THE FIBRE-DEFICIENT GUT

Our 21st-century diet deprives us of the most important nutrient of all: fibre. Dietary guidelines in the UK and the US recommend that adults eat a minimum of 30g of fibre each day. The vast majority of adults do not achieve this target, and virtually no-one eats the even higher fibre diet which the human digestive tract and microbiome have evolved to thrive on. (170-173) Fibre-deficiency can lead to bloating, indigestion, abdominal pain and troublesome bowel habits, symptoms that are incredibly common and severely affect more than one in ten adults. When these gut health symptoms begin to impact on quality of life, doctors often apply a diagnosis of irritable bowel syndrome (IBS). Although its often labelled as 'nothing serious', IBS can have a major impact on your quality of life. (174-176)

At just 38 years of age Emma had already accumulated a long list of medical diagnoses: type 2 diabetes, endometriosis, adhesions and polycystic ovarian syndrome. Her GP referred her to my clinic with severe digestive symptoms and added a new diagnosis to her list: 'severe IBS'. Various painkillers, medications to prevent cramps and simple laxatives had been tried without success. After multiple scans, endoscopies, blood tests and even exploratory abdominal surgery, Emma had been reassured that there was 'nothing seriously wrong'. But daily life was becoming almost impossible. On one occasion her bloating and pain were so severe that she had found herself in the emergency department of her local hospital.

When I first met Emma at my clinic we started with the basics. My standard three questions (see page 13) revealed that she was eating a fibre-deficient diet. Like many people, she believed that all carbohydrates cause weight gain. She avoided wholegrains almost completely and never ate fruit. She liked vegetables and aimed to eat two or three servings per day. It was time to bring in the plants! We agreed to some fibre-focused changes. She would eat three servings of wholegrains per day, begin to snack on whole fruits and opt for healthy, plant-based sources of protein whenever possible. Given the severity of her symptoms, I recommended one more test: an MRI scan of her bowel.

Emma came to her three-month follow-up appointment with her husband. They were both smiling as they walked into my office. Happily, the MRI scan had come back all clear. I talked her through the results. She pretended to be interested in the pictures but obviously had something more important to discuss. After three months of actively correcting her fibre deficiency her 'severe IBS' had resolved entirely. She'd also experienced healthy weight loss without counting calories and had much better control of

her type 2 diabetes. She was finding her blood sugars far easier to manage and her HbA1c blood test (which measures control of diabetes) had improved from 68 to 50 mmol/l. Her husband had been alongside her every step of the way and they were both thriving. Consultations like this make my day. I can't blame Emma for her previous fibre-deficient approach to food. She'd been doing her best with the information that was available. In a world of confusing media reports and a food culture that promotes processed convenience foods over fresh wholefoods and scares people away from eating even healthy carbohydrates, an unhealthy low-fibre diet has become the norm.

Patients with severe digestive health symptoms like Emma's should always discuss their symptoms with their doctor and ask whether a referral to a specialist is needed. Like many of the conditions I treat, there is often more than one cause. Genetic factors, problems with bile salt metabolism, difficulties with the gut–brain axis, personal and emotional stress, and negative changes in the gut microbiome have all been implicated in causing IBS. (177) However, given the importance of fibre and plants to gut health, it doesn't surprise me that 'irritable bowel syndrome' is so common in countries that have embraced the fibre-deficient Standard Western Diet. (178)

Cancer risk: the less meat and the more plants, the better.

One of the most difficult parts of my job is when I sit down with a patient to explain a new diagnosis of bowel cancer. I'm constantly in awe of people's resilience when faced with such devastating news. After each encounter I reflect on the fact that almost 1.5 million people around the globe have the same life-changing conversation with their doctor each year. (179) Bowel cancer is the UK's fourth leading cancer diagnosis, striking 1 in 15 men and 1 in 18 women in their lifetime. (180) But it is almost unknown among some rural populations. (181) The disparity could be due to many factors: cigarettes, alcohol, antibiotic use, environmental toxins or some other aspects of urban life that we don't even know about. But what about the role of diet?

The connection between eating meat and developing bowel cancer has been known for decades. In the 1990s researchers followed cancer rates in a group of almost 89,000 healthy middle-aged women. (182) Over just six years, women who ate red meat daily were 2.5 times more likely to develop bowel cancer than women who ate red meat less than once a month. Completely avoiding red meat reduced the risk by 60%. The latest data from the UK bears this out. Having followed almost half a million people for six years, the UK Biobank research team found that eating just one serving of red meat a day is linked with an 18% boost in bowel cancer risk. (183) Eating more plants, especially grains and cereals, reduces the risk significantly. The less meat and the more plants, the better. (184) In fact, eating a high-vegetable, low-meat diet may reduce your chances of bowel cancer by a factor of eight. (185)

There are many substances in cooked meat that could cause cancer: haem iron, heterocyclic amines, poly-cyclic aromatic polycarbons, nitrates and nitrites have all been implicated. (186-190) The evidence linking bacon, sausages, cured meats and other processed meats to bowel cancer is so convincing that in 2015 the World Health Organization listed these foods as 'Group 1 carcinogens: known to cause cancer in humans'. Other Group 1 carcinogens include cigarette smoke and asbestos. I'm patiently awaiting the day when this warning is clearly printed on packets of bacon! (191, 192)

How to avoid a 'carcinogenic gut microbiome'

Our gut microbiome plays a major role in how food influences our risk of bowel cancer. In 2019, *Nature*, the world's leading science journal, published two deep dives into the microbiome and cancer. (193, 194) These papers were impressive, combining data from multiple studies examining the complex interactions between gut bugs and health. Comparing bowel cancer patients to healthy individuals, they found definite microbiome signatures associated with cancer. These signatures were consistent in multiple populations and multiple countries. The microbiomes of cancer patients were substantially enriched with the bacteria that thrive on meat and fat. The results: a higher capacity to produce secondary bile acids, which are known carcinogens, and to convert choline (from eggs) and carnitine (from meat) into trimethylamine, a substance that promotes inflammation. Unsurprisingly, the bacteria that digest fruits, vegetables and wholegrains were markedly lower in cancer cases. The carcinogenic microbiome could well be described as the Standard Western Diet microbiome.

The authors of both papers were so struck by these differences that they proposed developing advanced microbiome analysis as a test for bowel cancer risk. It makes sense, right? If you have a lot of meat-loving and egg-loving bacteria, maybe you should be tested for cancer? But why wait for fancy new tests? We know that you can reduce and even eradicate these harmful gut bugs by switching to a healthy, plant-based diet. Making the switch from the Standard Western Diet to a whole-food, plant-based diet can dramatically cut your risk of developing bowel cancer in a matter of weeks. (195)

Bowel cancer remains a common diagnosis and is becoming more so, with rates tripling in younger Europeans since 1990. This is not due to rare genetic syndromes or bad luck, but to rising rates of obesity and poor dietary habits. (196) Cancer Research UK estimates that 12,000 people in the UK develop bowel cancer each year simply through eating a low-fibre diet, and a further 9,000 cases occur from eating red and processed meat. (197) There's a lot you can do to vastly reduce your risk: don't smoke, keep alcohol to a minimum and ask your doctor about screening. If you have symptoms, tell someone and get checked. Choosing a diet built from a rich variety of plants ticks all the right boxes to reduce your overall risk, and may also offer significant protection against cancers of the breast, prostate, stomach and pancreas. (198-217) In 2020, the doctors, dieticians, epidemiologists, and public health professionals of the American Cancer Society described a healthy cancer-preventing diet as follows (359):

'A healthy eating pattern includes foods that are high in nutrients in amounts that help achieve and maintain a healthy body weight; a variety of vegetables – dark green, red, and orange, fibre-rich legumes (beans and peas), and other vegetables; fruits, especially whole fruits with a variety of colours; and wholegrains.'

I can't think of a better description of a whole-food, plant-based diet!

> Choosing a diet built from a rich variety of plants ticks all the right boxes to reduce your overall risk, and may also offer significant protection against cancers of the breast, prostate, stomach and pancreas.

FERMENTED FOODS: NATURE'S MICROBIOME BOOST?

Plant-based fermented foods have been around since the dawn of human civilisation. With recent appreciation of their taste profiles and potential health benefits, fermented foods like tempeh, miso and kimchi are back on the menu. The recipes for Tempeh miso stir-fry and Sticky tofu, courgettes, greens & kimchi (see pages 142 and 146) show you just how much flavour these fermented foods can bring to your plate. The ancient techniques used to produce them take advantage of the ability of bacterial cultures to break down and ferment foods, radically changing their taste and flavour profile. Fermented foods can contain dozens or even hundreds of bacterial strains. They often contain more than 1 million live bacteria per gram. (218) Most fermented foods have a predominance of lactic acid bacteria, which love digesting fibre to generate beneficial compounds such as short-chain fatty acids.

Numerous studies have suggested that fermented foods may have unique health benefits. For example, eating a daily serving of kimchi improved glucose control and improved insulin sensitivity in volunteers with pre-diabetes. (219) Other researchers have suggested that fermented soy products can help to reduce body fat and improve cholesterol. (220) Although fermented plant-based foods contain many of the same bacterial species that are sold as probiotic supplements, there haven't been many studies on the effects that fermented foods have on our gut health. (221) More research is needed. In the meantime, I enjoy fermented foods as an occasional tasty and interesting addition to my plant-based diet, with some potential side-benefits for my gut microbiome. If you don't enjoy their complex flavours, don't worry. Kimchi and sauerkraut are not considered essential to a healthy plant-based diet. Besides which, many raw fruits and vegetables naturally provide the very same beneficial bacteria that are found in fermented foods. (222)

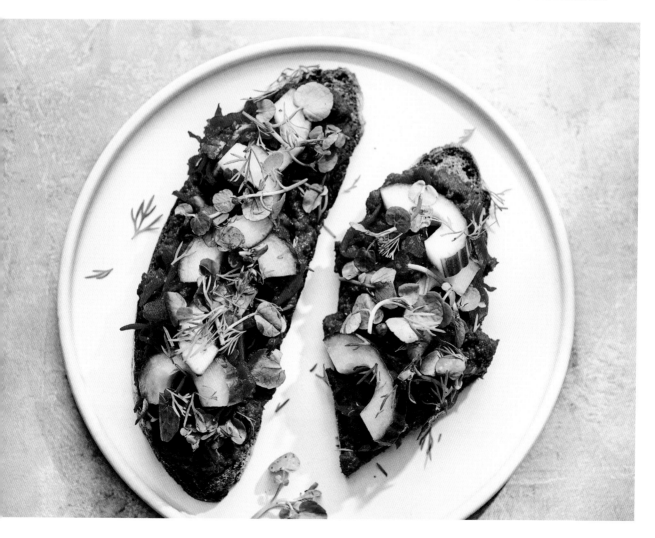

HEALTHY HEART

Food is deeply important to us. No matter how busy our day, most of us wake up in the morning looking forward to our breakfast and soon begin planning what we'll have for lunch. Dinner marks the end of the daytime rush and is often the first chance to sit and catch up with friends and family. Birthdays, weddings and reunions... whenever we celebrate, there is a special meal to be shared. The meals we eat help us to define our identity and our culture. We even have 'national' dishes. Food is also one of the main drivers of our health and longevity. Food is powerful. It can even prevent our number one killer: cardiovascular disease.

Cardiovascular disease is the number one cause of death in high-income countries like the UK, Ireland and USA. (223, 224) Heart attacks, strokes, high blood pressure and related conditions claim 17.8 million lives globally per year. These diseases are so common that we have come to view them as normal. By the time we reach the age of 70, we almost expect that we'll be on a list of medications to keep our blood pressure and cholesterol under control. But it doesn't have to be like this. These conditions are not inevitable; they are not a normal part of the ageing process. By choosing a plant-focused diet and a healthy lifestyle, you can drastically reduce your risk of cardiovascular disease and add good years to your life. Years without chest pain, breathlessness, cardiac stents and without by-pass surgery. Cardiovascular disease may be our number one killer, but most cases can be prevented. (225–227)

START WITH THE FOOD ON YOUR PLATE

In 2019 the American College of Cardiology issued their official guidelines on how to protect our cardiac health. (228) Their advice on diet was simple. The more animal products on your plate, the higher your risk. The more plants on your plate, the lower your risk. (228-235) To quote the American Heart Association: 'Whether you're considering eating less meat or giving it up entirely, the benefits are clear: less risk of disease and improved health and well-being'. (236)

To better understand the impact that food has on heart health, let's look at one of world's healthiest populations. The Seventh Day Adventists of Loma Linda, California, are widely recognised as one of the longest-lived communities on the planet. (237) In many ways, they have figured out the secrets to a longer and healthier life and built them into their everyday practices. Most Seventh Day Adventists don't smoke. They also exercise regularly, make sure to spend time in nature and value connections with their families and communities. As part of their dedication to health, they take a plant-based approach to food. About half the Adventist population are vegetarian and 1 in 12 eat a completely plant-based diet. (238) Those who do eat meat have it in small amounts, just four servings per week. (239) Thanks to their healthier approach to diet and lifestyle, the Seventh Day Adventists have reduced their risk of heart disease by an impressive 50%. (240) Amongst this mostly vegetarian population, those who eat a completely-plant based diet decrease their risk even further. (241, 242)

By eating meat, eggs and dairy we get our calories wrapped up in a package of cholesterol and saturated fat, which are both potent drivers of the disease processes that lead to heart disease. By contrast, calories obtained from plants come packaged with the fibre, healthy fats, antioxidants, vitamins, minerals and phytochemicals that keep our hearts healthy. If you eat red or processed meat each day, replacing it calorie for calorie with nuts, legumes or wholegrains can cut your risk of heart disease by up to 47%. (243)

FIVE HEART-HEALTHY HABITS THAT EVERYONE SHOULD KNOW

In 2014 Swedish researchers identified five healthy habits that could make you virtually immune to heart disease. (244)

1. Eat a diet that maximises your intake of fruits, vegetables, wholegrains, nuts and legumes (you probably guessed that one!).

2. Avoid excess alcohol. If you do drink, limit your intake to 1-3 standard drinks per day.

3. Never smoke (and if you do, quit now).

4. Get some exercise. Ideally you should break a sweat for 40 minutes each day.

5. Maintain a healthy body weight with a waist measurement of less than 97cm (37 inches).

Having followed 20,000 volunteers for over a decade, the researchers found that just two of these five habits reduced the risk of having a heart attack by 36%. That's impressive. But volunteers with the healthiest diet plus all of the other four habits did much better, reducing their risk by up to 93%. When it comes to preventing our number one killer, a very healthy diet and lifestyle beats moderation hands down!

'Whether you're considering eating less meat or giving it up entirely, the benefits are clear: less risk of disease and improved health and well-being.'

THE AMERICAN HEART ASSOCIATION

STOPPING HEART DISEASE IN ITS TRACKS

In 2014 Dr Caldwell Esselstyn Jr and his colleges published the experience of patients attending their practice at the world-famous Cleveland Clinic. (245) They had followed up almost 200 patients at risk of cardiovascular disease, all of whom had received counselling on adapting to a whole-food, plant-based diet. Among the patients who disregarded their advice and decided to continue with the diet and lifestyle that had brought them to the clinic in the first place, almost two-thirds went on to experience a heart attack or stroke. Gladly, the majority of Dr Esselstyn's patients stuck to the plant-based plan. The rate of further serious cardiovascular events among those who adapted the recommended dietary change was less than 1%. The success of Dr Esselstyn's programme showed the true power of a healthy diet and lifestyle, proving that even established heart disease can be stopped in its tracks.

Choosing to get your protein from plants may be one of the best decisions you can make to protect your heart health. The animal products that are known to drive heart disease in each country vary, depending on the national diet. In the US it's red and processed meat, in Japan it's fish and in Holland it's meat and dairy. Whatever country you live in, switching out animal products for more plants on your plate will significantly increase your chances of a life without heart disease. (246)

YOUR BODY MAKES ALL THE CHOLESTEROL YOU NEED

Cholesterol is a fatty substance that is manufactured by your liver and travels around your body in your bloodstream. Your body needs this cholesterol for multiple essential tasks. It's an important component of the membranes that enclose every single cell in your body and it is used to manufacture crucial hormones and fat-soluble vitamins. Cholesterol is also used to make bile, without which you could not effectively digest many foods. Cholesterol is essential to your health and well-being. Which is why your body makes it.

If you have too much cholesterol in your bloodstream, it can accumulate in the walls of your blood vessels. This process, called 'atherosclerosis', narrows the blood vessels and reduces the blood supply to vital organs, including your heart and your brain. By keeping your blood cholesterol level in the healthy range, you prevent atherosclerosis and significantly reduce your risk of ever suffering a heart attack or a stroke. (246)

Here's the key point: your body makes all the cholesterol you need. You have no biological need to get extra cholesterol by eating chickens, cows, pigs or any other animal. The more cholesterol you eat, the more cholesterol in your bloodstream and the higher your risk of heart disease. (247) A plant-based diet maximises your chances of keeping your cholesterol in the healthy range. You'll understand why by looking at the list opposite, which shows the cholesterol content of some popular foods.

FOOD	CHOLESTEROL PER 100G (4OZ) SERVING
Chicken	86mg
Salmon	75mg
Pork	72mg
Lean beef	62mg
Cashew nuts	zero
Beans	zero
Avocado	zero
Brown rice	zero

That's right, plants do not contain cholesterol. No matter how much you eat, every item on your plant-powered plate contains zero cholesterol per serving!

THE SOUTH-WEST PLANT-BASED DIET CHALLENGE

In January 2020 I challenged 100 health professionals in the South West of England to start their own health revolution by going plant-based for 28 days. Before the challenge, nobody in the group was eating a whole food, plant-based diet. I promised that four weeks of eating delicious meals with no calorie counting would lead to healthy weight loss and impressive reductions in their cholesterol. I joined forces with my friends, plant-based chefs Stephen and David Flynn of the Happy Pear, and a team of local volunteers. We provided all the tools our challengers needed to achieve these goals: recipes and meal plans just like the ones in this book, as well as pot-luck lunchtime meet-ups, live cooking demonstrations and educational events. Challengers even joined us for a sunrise swim in the sea (quickly followed by warming bowls of porridge and mugs of hot coffee!).

Almost half of our sign-ups were doctors. They were joined by a mix of other front-line health professionals: nurses, pharmacists, dietitians, physiotherapists and administrative staff. One-third started the challenge with elevated non-HDL cholesterol levels, a strong predictor of future heart disease or stroke. After just four weeks of eating as much cholesterol-free food as they liked, their harmful cholesterol levels had dropped by an average of 27%. By the end of the South West Plant-Based Diet Challenge, 94% of the group had cholesterol levels firmly in the heart-healthy range. Challengers who'd been living with obesity or overweight had also seen an average weight loss of 5kg. Over the 28 days, many of these health-care professionals had moved into the healthy body weight bracket for the first time in years.

My colleagues were impressed. They had lost weight, dropped their cholesterol and substantially reduced their risk of developing heart disease. (248, 249) As medical professionals, they knew that results like these can be difficult to achieve with medications. Their numbers were exciting, but for me the major result was the culture change that the challenge sparked. These doctors and health professionals had heard me speaking about why I recommend a plant-based diet to my patients, but for them, those benefits had been theoretical at best. Many entered the challenge with a fair degree of scepticism. In just one month they'd learned that plant-based meals are delicious and seen dramatic health benefits for themselves. Almost three-quarters of the group decided to make the switch to a plant-based diet permanently. Even those who went back to eating animal products vastly reduced the amount on their plate. Since the challenge I've been working with my (now enthusiastic) colleagues to find ways of bringing these same plant-powered benefits to more of the people who need them the most: our patients.

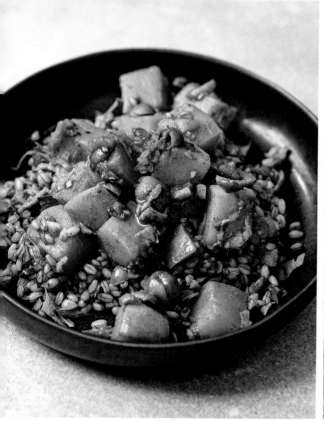
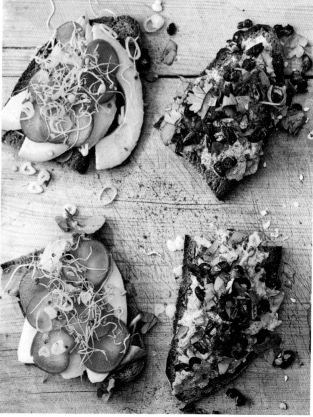

HOW TO FIX YOUR BLOOD PRESSURE WITH PLANTS

The blood vessels that run through your body are part of a system that is kept flowing by your beating heart. We can measure how much of the heart's pumping pressure is transmitted through your blood vessels by putting a cuff around your arm and taking your blood pressure or 'BP'. Keeping that BP at a healthy number seriously increases your chances of avoiding heart disease, kidney failure and stroke. (250) Here are two things you can do to stop yours from rising.

FIRST, CUT THE SALT. The more salt in your diet, the more salt in your body. To dilute that salt, your body absorbs more water. More fluid in the system drives the pressure up. Reducing the salt in your diet isn't simply a matter of adding less to your food at home. Just 18% of dietary salt comes from the extra we sprinkle on while cooking or when we sit down to eat. In the UK, 61% of dietary salt comes from the salt already added to processed foods and a further 21% comes from the salt naturally present in foods. The main sources of the salt in our diet? Breakfast cereals, meat products, ready-made meals and dairy products including cheese. (251-253) By preparing your own plant-based meals you'll be cutting your salt intake dramatically.

SECOND, ADD THE PLANTS. Fruits, nuts, pulses, leafy greens, oats and berries each have unique properties that will keep your blood pressure under control. (254-256) This is not just about adding fibre! Plants like beetroot, spinach, radishes, lettuce and celery are also rich sources of nitrates, chemicals that improve blood flow and reduce the pressure in the system. (257)

Just like high cholesterol, high blood pressure should not be regarded as a normal part of the aging process. By filling your diet with a rich diversity of plants you can keep both at a healthy number for decades to come.

> Keeping that BP at a healthy number seriously increases your chances of avoiding heart disease, kidney failure and stroke.

PLANT-BASED SUCCESS: ANDY'S STORY

Heart disease can sneak up on you. At 35 years of age, my friend Andy Ramage was surprised to find himself in a cardiologist's office. As a former professional footballer, Andy was used to being the fittest guy in the room. However, over the years of building a career as a senior broker at a high-powered London firm, he'd seen his health and fitness decline. In his own words he was 'a lifelong salad dodger, three stone overweight, incredibly unhealthy, stressed out and maxed out'.

Andy had just had a coronary calcium scan, checking for atherosclerosis, the furring of the arteries that causes heart disease. The cardiologist, Dr Gupta, warned him that the results were not good: Andy already had significant heart disease. He decided to take control of his health. Having read as many reliable resources as he could find, he gave his life a plant-based overhaul. Food would become the fuel for his recovery.

Two years later, thanks to a whole-food, plant-based diet, the decision to quit alcohol and a renewed fitness routine, things had improved dramatically. Andy checked back in with Dr Gupta. 'The results were staggering. I looked like a different person. I had gone from looking like Homer Simpson on a bad day to, well, me 15 years younger!'

'Astounding!' said Dr Gupta. 'Your resting heart rate has plummeted from 67 to 42, your bad cholesterol is fantastic at 2.7mmol/L [104mg/dl in US units], your blood pressure is lower, you're 19kg [42lb] lighter and you look great. But what's really amazing is that it appears you have stopped your heart disease.' At this point he called in his colleague and continued, 'In fact, we both believe you have reversed it!'

Andy's story is truly inspiring. Having transformed his health by changing his diet and lifestyle for the better, Andy soon forged a successful career as an author and motivational coach.

THE MICROBIOME-HEART CONNECTION

In 2017 an international team of researchers announced that a new blood test could identify patients at risk of heart disease. They'd measured blood levels of this new biomarker in 500 patients who'd attended the emergency department with a suspected heart attack. Patients with the highest levels were far more likely to go on to have a major cardiac event. (258) Further research has shown this blood test also works outside the emergency room. Even in healthy individuals, an elevated level is a risk factor for future heart disease. (259-260) The substance they were checking for is called trimethylamine N-oxide (TMAO). Where does it come from? It's made by your gut microbiome when you eat meat or eggs.

Specific gut bacteria metabolise meat and eggs to produce a chemical called TMA (just like healthy bacteria convert fibre into SCFA). The TMA is then absorbed by your gut lining and transported to the liver, which turns it into TMAO, a pro-inflammatory molecule that enters the bloodstream and accelerates the formation of the fatty plaques in the arteries that cause heart disease. This harmful chemical, produced by the meat- and egg-fed microbiome, has also been linked to causing chronic kidney damage and may even increase your risk of having a stroke. (261, 262)

New drugs to block the microbiome bacteria that make this harmful compound are already being developed by the pharmaceutical industry. The good news is that you don't need medications to enjoy the benefits of a heart-healthy gut microbiome. You can flatten your TMAO levels and your risk of heart disease right now by making the switch to a whole-food, plant-based diet. (263-264)

In 2019 researchers asked 26 healthy volunteers to try 3 popular weight-loss diets, sticking carefully to each one for 4 weeks. The high-fat Atkins diet (which allows lots of meat and eggs but very few fruits and vegetables), the high protein South Beach diet (which allows lean meats plus fruits and vegetables), and a whole-food, plant-based diet. For this experiment everybody's calories were adjusted regularly to make sure that they did not lose weight. The researchers were far more interested in what happened to their TMAO levels. (264)

On the Atkins diet and the South Beach diet, volunteers were feeding their microbes plenty of meat and eggs. They recorded rapid and significant boosts in TMAO production. The whole-food, plant-based diet had the opposite effect. As the bacteria needed to metabolise meat and eggs died off, levels of this harmful biomarker reduced significantly. In just 28 days the study participants had harnessed the power of their gut microbiome to protect them from one of our most common diseases. This short-term study shows that the gut microbiome is a crucial player in the outcome we see time and again in long-term population studies: a diet based on animal products increases your risk of heart disease. If you know someone who would like to achieve a healthier body weight, please steer them away from Dr Atkins and towards the plant-based diet revolution. This approach will ensure that they meet their goals while keeping their heart, gut and microbiome in excellent health!

'In less than six months of eating a plant-based diet my total cholesterol has come down dramatically. I've never been overweight and have always been active. I thought my diet was good. Please, please tell all your patients.'

MESSAGE RECEIVED VIA INSTAGRAM

HEALTHY BODY

_____

In 2019 Norwegian researchers published a fascinating study that had taken over half a century to complete. With data collection that started in the 1960s, they charted obesity rates among 120,000 healthy adults over a 50-year period. (265) They also performed genetic analysis on participants to find out how strongly their genes influenced their weight gain. In the 1960s people with the most 'obesity genes' had only a 1 in 10 chance of actually becoming obese. By 2008 their chances had risen to almost 1 in 3. As you'd expect, the individuals with no genetic predisposition to weight gain tended to maintain a healthy body weight. But by the 21st century more than 1 in 8 of even the most 'genetically thin' adults were also living with obesity. When it comes to body weight, our diet and lifestyle are far more important factors than the genes that we inherit from our parents and ancestors.

Our current lifestyles seem to be designed for lifelong weight gain – the calorie-laden Standard Western Diet, endless hours of screen time and towns that are designed for cars and not people – these all contribute to the modern 'obesogenic environment'. Global obesity rates have tripled since 1975, and right now two-thirds of Western adults are living with excess weight or obesity. (266) The good news is that you can escape this trend. A plant-based approach to food might even make you immune to the global epidemic of excess weight gain. (267)

Maintaining a healthy body weight has multiple long-term benefits, not least far lower risks of heart disease, stroke and multiple cancers, which in turn mean improved chances of a longer, happier and disease-free life. (268–271) The fat cells that accumulate due to obesity are metabolically active and help to keep your body in a state of low-grade inflammation. For example, excess fat deposited within the liver causes a condition called fatty liver disease. In its more aggressive forms, this pro-inflammatory condition causes permanent liver damage. Living in an obesogenic environment, an incredible 1 in 5 young adults in the UK now has fatty liver disease. (272) This preventable condition is soon expected to become our number one reason for needing a liver transplant. (273) To avoid and even reverse the build-up of pro-inflammatory fat in your liver, the more whole-food and plant-based your diet, the better. (274, 275)

A PRESCRIPTION TO EAT MORE PLANTS

Back in 1998, when I was halfway through medical school, Dr Hans Diehl published the results of a successful community health initiative that he'd launched in Kalamazoo, Michigan. (276) He enrolled 304 local residents in a one-month programme to improve their well-being. His participants needed it – some 70% were overweight or obese, one-third already had heart disease, and almost half had high blood pressure. This was a healthy-eating programme with a difference. There would be no calorie counting and no portion control. Instead, participants learned to prepare meals based on the 'optimal diet': beans, greens, wholegrains, legumes, fresh fruits and vegetables. Trips to the gym were not required, but participants were encouraged to walk or exercise for just 30 minutes each day.

After four weeks the results were impressive. Eating as much food as they liked and walking about 3km (2 miles) per day, the group lost an average 2.7kg (6lb) in body weight. Alongside healthy weight loss, the volunteers achieved significant reductions in high cholesterol and blood pressure. Dr Diehl and his colleagues went on to repeat this success in dozens of communities, and published over 40 research papers demonstrating the long-term effectiveness of what has become known as the Complete Health Improvement Programme (276) – a whole-food, plant-based intervention that achieves and maintains a healthier body.

You'll notice that the Recipes for the Revolution and the 28-Day Revolution meal plans do not include calorie counts. As you embark on your plant-based diet revolution, your focus will be on the quality of your food, rather than the quantity. Building your meals with fruits, vegetables, beans, greens and wholegrains while eating to your natural appetite means that just like Dr Diehl's very first volunteers, you will effortlessly consume fewer calories and more of the nutrients that will help you to achieve and maintain a healthy body weight. No counting required. (276-280)

FOODS THAT BURN MORE CALORIES

The main determinant of how many calories you burn in a day isn't the amount of food you eat or how many hours you spend in the gym. It's your basal metabolic rate. This is how many calories you use just to keep your body ticking along. Standing, sitting, thinking, digesting food, breathing, pumping blood around your body, building muscle and growing your hair – all these processes use up calories. The average male burns about 1,800 calories a day, and the average female about 1,400 calories, by doing nothing at all! If you could increase that metabolic number, you would lose weight without even trying. A plant-based diet does just that, boosting your resting metabolism by 10–20%. (281-283) Over weeks and months this can add up to thousands of additional calories burned by simply eating more plants. This may be one of the main reasons that people who eat a plant-based diet are far less likely to be overweight or obese. (284)

THE MORE CARBS YOU EAT, THE BETTER

The statement that 'healthy carbs help you to lose weight' sounds controversial, but by now it should not surprise you. 'Healthy carbs' is really just another way of saying 'whole plants'. The evidence: doctors randomised 75 overweight American adults to either a whole-food, plant-based diet or their standard diet for 16 weeks. There was no calorie counting and no limits set on portion size. During the 16 weeks volunteers were very carefully monitored for dietary intake, body weight and body composition.

The group who continued as before did not lose weight – no surprise there! But the plant-based group lost an average of 6.5kg (14lb), of which 4.3kg (9½lb) was fat. Statistical analysis showed that the more carbohydrates they consumed, the better their results. On the plan, 70% of calories came from complex carbohydrates, including wholegrains, legumes, fruits and vegetables. These are fibre-rich foods which increase feelings of satiety, promote a healthy microbiome, reduce appetite and aid blood sugar regulation by multiple mechanisms. This study proved that effective weight loss does not require a low-carb, high-meat diet; in fact, the opposite is true. When the plan is whole-food and plant-based, motivated people can stick with the programme and achieve great results. (285)

INSULIN RESISTANCE AND TYPE 2 DIABETES

Obesity is intricately linked to one of our most common chronic illnesses: type 2 diabetes. People with this condition have become resistant to the effects of their own body's insulin. This results in high blood sugars (hyperglycaemia), a state that promotes atherosclerosis, the furring of the arteries that causes heart disease. Type 2 diabetes also leads to kidney damage and increased risk of stroke and blindness. In the long term, the damage caused by having high blood sugar even reduces the body's ability to produce insulin in the first place. Since 1980 the number of people in the world with type 2 diabetes has more than quadrupled. (286) In the UK, 1 in 10 people over 40 now live with this condition, many of them requiring multiple medications and daily insulin injections to try to control their blood sugars and slow the damage to their health. (287-288)

So how should we eat to prevent type 2 diabetes? We've known for decades that food, obesity and insulin resistance are strongly linked. When Dutch researchers followed 7,000 adults for 8 years their verdict was clear: those with the highest 'plant-based dietary index' were the least likely to develop insulin resistance or type 2 diabetes. (289) To explain these findings the researchers pointed to the multiple known benefits of a whole-food, plant-based diet: higher intake of fibre, antioxidants and plant-based oils, all of which contribute to a healthier body weight, improved responsiveness to high blood sugars, reduced inflammation and lower cholesterol. By contrast, animal products provide the saturated fats, animal proteins and pro-inflammatory molecules that impair glucose metabolism and make the body resistant to the effects of insulin. (290-297) The link between eating meat and developing type 2 diabetes shows a clear 'dose-response' relationship. The more meat you eat, the more likely the disease. Adding just 100g (4oz) of meat (or half a large burger patty) to your plate each day may increase your chances of developing type 2 diabetes by up to 49%. (298)

While eating more plants and less meat is protective, data from the Seventh Day Adventist population (see page 39) suggest that a completely plant-based diet may be even more powerful. The Adventist Health Study 2 followed over 40,000 adults for two years. (299) During the study period, type 2 diabetes was diagnosed in 1 in 47 meat-eating Adventists. But a fully plant-based diet reduced the risk to 1 in 185. When statistical methods were used to remove age, gender, educational level, income, physical activity, alcohol, smoking and body weight from the calculations, a completely plant-based diet alone was estimated to cut the risk of developing diabetes by an impressive 62%. That's a huge number.

THE FRUIT AND VEGETABLE TEST

Studies that examine the long-term impact of eating fruits and vegetables usually ask volunteers to fill out food diaries and then follow their health outcomes for years. Although researchers use carefully designed questionnaires and may even ask volunteers to photograph all their meals for a few days, these studies can never be 100% accurate. It's human nature. No one wants to look bad in front of a food researcher! It's well known that when asked 'what did you eat today?' some volunteers are likely to add a few extra apples or forget to include the bacon sandwich with extra cheese they had for breakfast. With large studies, these inaccuracies get ironed out, but wouldn't it be wonderful if researchers could use a reliable 'fruit and vegetable test', a blood test that would tell them exactly how much fruit and veg their volunteers were really eating?

A European-wide research team recently did exactly this, measuring blood levels of plant-derived nutrients – including vitamin C, carotenoids and lycopene – in 23,000 volunteers across 8 different countries. (300) The results were clear. The more plant-based nutrients in their bloodstream, the less likely they were to develop type 2 diabetes. Volunteers whose test results put them in the top 20% of the population for eating fruits and vegetables cut their personal risk of developing type 2 diabetes by half. By taking human nature out of the equation, these researchers demonstrated that healthy food choices are even more powerful than we'd previously thought.

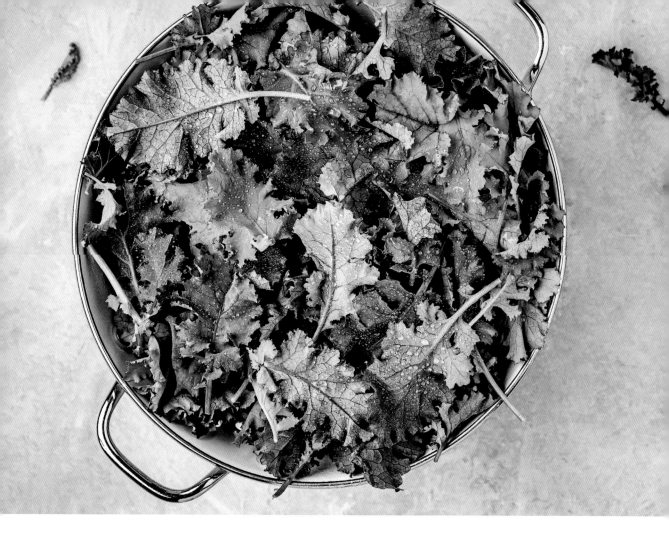

THE POWER OF A PLANT-FUELLED MICROBIOME

Our gut microbes play a key role in preventing and reversing type 2 diabetes. When researchers randomly assigned volunteers with this diagnosis to eat either a balanced omnivorous diet or a whole-food, plant-based diet (including nine wholegrains, beans, oats, corn and some nuts), the differences in response were impressive. (301) With 38g of fibre a day, the plant-based group showed rapid and significant benefits in gut microbial diversity. Within 28 days their microbes were changing to produce significantly more beneficial short-chain fatty acids (SCFAs, see page 30). In theory, boosting SCFA production should help to control blood sugars and reduce appetite – and that's exactly what happened. Subjects on the plant-based diet lost 4.2% of their body weight and achieved excellent diabetic control in 90% of cases. Disease reversal! The omnivorous group ate the same overall calories and macronutrients, but included meat, eggs and dairy in their diet. Fewer plants meant less fibre, just

16g per day. Only half of this group achieved diabetic control, and the average weight loss was just 1.5% of body weight.

What the researchers did next confirmed the power of a plant-fuelled microbiome. When they administered a microbiome transplant from the study participants to laboratory mice, those mice that received a plant-based microbiome immediately showed improved blood sugar control. Having identified 4.8 million microbiome genes, they narrowed down the beneficial effects to just 15 bacterial strains that thrived in the high-fibre environment. Am I recommending that you take a probiotic supplement containing those 15 fibre-loving bacteria? Or that you convince someone to give you a microbiome transplant from a donor who already eats a healthy plant-based diet? Nope. I just want you to maximise the plants on your plate three times a day!

CAN A PLANT-BASED DIET REVERSE METABOLIC SYNDROME?

Obesity, high cholesterol and type 2 diabetes occur together so often that there is a medical term to describe all three in combination: metabolic syndrome. A key driver of this syndrome is the Standard Western Diet. In 2013 a team of South Korean researchers decided to test if the reverse was true. (302) Could a whole-food, plant-based diet reverse all three major components of metabolic syndrome?

Six obese volunteers with metabolic syndrome were placed on a healthy and completely plant-based diet for one month. On their new meal plan their daily fibre intake was 42g and they were getting almost three-quarters of their calories from whole carbohydrates. In just 28 days they lost an average 10% of their starting body weight. They also markedly improved control of their type 2 diabetes and dropped their cholesterol back into the normal range. Changes in their gut microbiome helped to explain these benefits.

In four weeks the researchers measured significant microbiome improvements, with harmful pro-inflammatory bacteria dying off and increased numbers of beneficial bacteria thriving. As they began to feed their healthy bacteria and reverse their metabolic syndrome, all participants also showed significant reductions in baseline levels of gut inflammation. This was a small study, but the results remain impressive, showing exactly how to kickstart healthy weight loss, lower cholesterol, improve diabetic control, reduce intestinal inflammation and generate beneficial shifts in the gut microbiome – all in just 28 days.

Advising patients with type 2 diabetes and metabolic syndrome to adopt a plant-based diet should not be viewed as a controversial treatment plan. The evidence showing that a plant-based diet is their best option is compelling. In 2019 the expert panel charged with writing the official US guidelines for the treatment of type 2 diabetes and obesity gave a clear recommendation based on decades of scientific evidence: 'All patients should strive to attain and maintain an optimal weight through a primarily plant-based meal plan.' (303)

PLANT-BASED SUCCESS: MATT'S STORY

Matt was 57 years old when he first came to see me at my clinic. His GP was worried. Routine blood tests had revealed abnormal liver function and significant inflammation. After further tests and a liver scan, the diagnosis was fatty liver disease. I explained that this was caused by food. Matt was not surprised. His job meant long hours behind the wheel of his car and he knew that his diet was 'not great'. He was eating less than two servings of fruits and vegetables a day. Processed meats, such as bacon, ham and sausages, were an almost daily event, and he described himself as a 'cheese fan'. He was clinically obese and well on his way to a diagnosis of type 2 diabetes. We agreed that things needed to change. With Matt's permission, here is an extract from the letter I wrote to his GP three months later:

I saw Matt for follow-up today regarding his non-alcoholic fatty liver disease. He is doing extremely well. On a whole-food, plant-based diet he continues to lose a healthy amount of weight. When I first met him three months ago, he weighed 114.1kg (251.5lb) with a BMI of 36. He is now down to 103.2kg (225lb) with a BMI of 32. For the first time in five years his HbA1C [measure of blood sugar level] is firmly within the normal range at 36, indicating that he no longer has pre-diabetes. His AST and ALT [tests for liver inflammation] continue to improve. Both he and his wife are very happy to continue with their revised dietary practices. I will see him back in two months.

Matt and his wife had assumed that he would live the rest of his life with pre-diabetes and gradually worsening health. We'd proved those assumptions wrong. At his next clinic visit, Matt weighed in at under 100kg (220lb). For the first time in many years, he was no longer classed as obese. As well as his impressive numbers, he'd discovered a new enthusiasm for cooking and was enjoying feeling healthier and more energetic every day. Consultations like these make it all worthwhile.

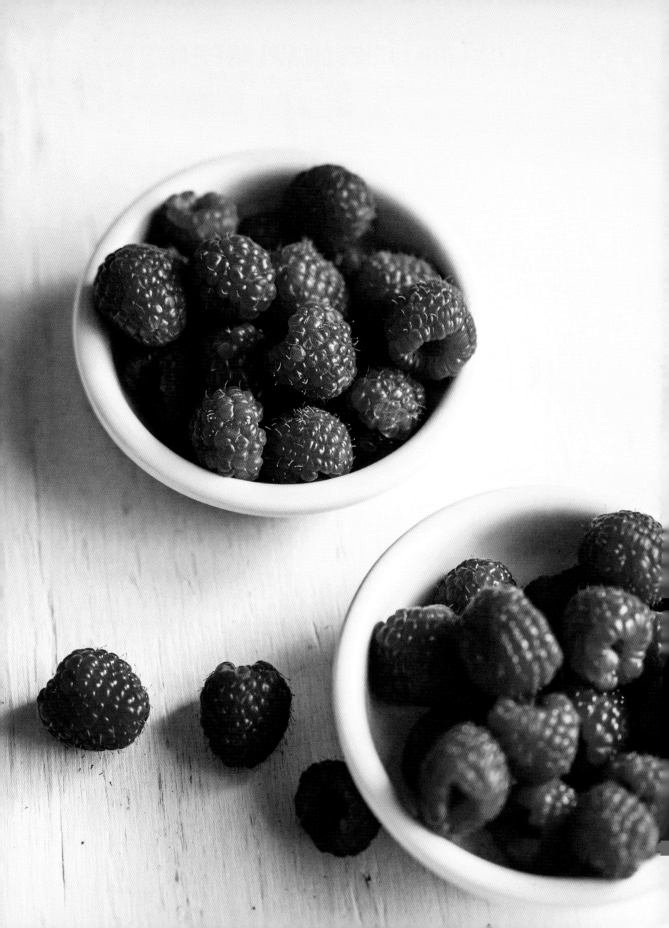

ATHLETES WHO THRIVE ON A PLANT-BASED DIET

A high-quality diet is a key requirement to becoming a successful athlete. Although many athletes focus almost exclusively on protein, this is just one aspect of an optimal diet. (304) As you now know, all plants contain protein. Even without meat, dairy or eggs, strict vegetarians consume an average 70g of protein per day and can hit 100g a day simply by eating more food. (305) A whole-food, plant-based diet holds many other advantages for high-performance athletes. The same benefits that improve blood flow to the heart and other vital organs, while reducing inflammation and helping maintain a healthy body weight, may also contribute to improved performance and recovery. (306)

As the plant-based diet revolution has continued its global spread, we've seen an increase in professional athletes making the change. Tennis champion Novak Djokovic, Formula One driver Lewis Hamilton, Rugby League player Anthony Mullally, Olympic cyclist Dotsie Bausch and World Cup-winning US National Women's Team footballer Alex Morgan are just a few of those who have spoken publicly about how a plant-based diet has helped them to achieve their athletic goals.

Despite the high-profile successes of plant-based athletes, many experts still maintain that a diet without meat, eggs and dairy could harm their athletic performance in the long term. In 2020, exercise science researchers at the University of Montreal decided to put this theory to the test, signing up 56 female athletes, all of who were non-smokers with a healthy body weight. (307) Half the volunteers were long-term vegans, the other half were lifelong consumers of meat, dairy and eggs. Physically, it was difficult for the sport scientists to tell if an athlete was vegan or not. Height, total body weight, body fat percentage, lean body mass and muscular strength did not differ between the two dietary groups. But once the athletes got on an exercise bike, the vegans were easier to spot. During intense exercise the plant-powered athletes showed that their muscles had a superior ability to utilise oxygen. On an exercise bike set at 70% of their maximum resistance and pedalling at 70–80 rpm for as long as they could, the omnivores managed an average 8.8 minutes before reaching the point of exhaustion. The plant-based athletes kept pedalling for an average of 12.2 minutes.

These high-performing athletes were eating a whole-food vegan diet, consuming 41g of fibre and 66g of plant-based protein per day. The researchers suggested that the advantages they recorded may have been due to better muscle glycogen stores, a higher intake of carbohydrates, or the known abilities of a plant-based diet to reduce oxidative stress and inflammation. Whatever the explanation, their conclusion was clear: 'Healthcare professionals should not discourage a vegan diet and may even want to consider it as an option during the implementation of an exercise training program.' Myth busted!

The foods you choose to fuel your body can be extremely powerful. As I've seen time and again in my clinic, a plant-based diet reduces inflammation, promotes healthy weight loss and can even reverse type 2 diabetes. The science suggests that it may even help to increase your athletic performance. When it comes to building a healthier body, it's plant-based all the way.

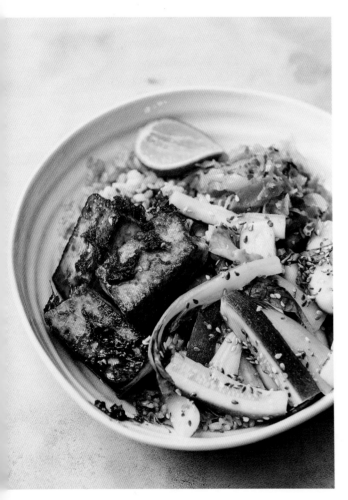

HOW TO BEAT THE OBESOGENIC ENVIRONMENT

In the 21st century our environment seems to be designed to promote excess weight gain. The most convenient foods are usually the unhealthiest, and many hours spent at desks, in front of screens or stuck in traffic also contribute to the problem. Here are five ways that you can fight back.

1 Make your own lunch. When you've made the effort to cook a delicious plant-based dinner, you deserve to enjoy it again. Cook more than you need and take the leftovers with you for tomorrow's lunch. Now you've had two home-cooked meals and avoided grabbing a less healthy option.

2 Get some secret exercise. Getting more active does not require a gym membership. Building physical activity into your day is cheaper and just as effective. Walking to the shops, vacuuming the house, standing at your desk, taking the stairs and playing with the kids all contribute to your daily calorie burn.

3 Shop local or shop online. If you have a local shop, it's a great excuse to make walking or biking part of your day. If you need to visit a large supermarket, try parking as far as you can from the entrance. Better still, order your shopping online for delivery. You'll avoid the impulse food purchases and can use the free time to take the neighbour's dog for a walk.

4 Spend more time with your healthiest friends. The people we see every day are a major influence on our attitudes and behaviours. Seek out your fittest friends and spend more time with them. If they are keen on early morning hiking trips, or pre-breakfast workouts, those may soon become a normal activity for you too.

5 Eat mindfully. It's tempting to use food as the solution to emotions that have nothing to do with hunger. When you find yourself reaching for a snack or treating yourself to an extra serving of dessert, try to pause and reflect on why. Are you really hungry? Or are you simply tired? Or bored? Eating unconsciously is a sure way to take on extra calories that your body simply does not need.

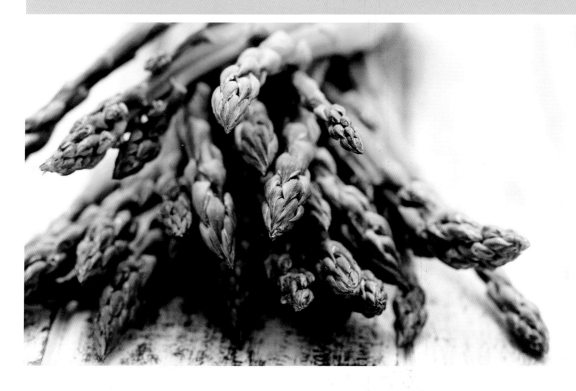

HEALTHY MIND

———

I've been privileged to help thousands of people make the change to a plant-based diet. Whether at my clinic, at public events, through online courses or during community plant-based challenges, there is one topic of conversation that keeps coming up: happiness. For example, Iona made the move to a whole-food, plant-based diet to improve her gut health. After one month she gave me this feedback:

> 'I feel more energetic, much lighter and more active. Happier, truly happier! It's just a fantastic result after four weeks.'

Lighter, more energetic and happier. Couldn't we all use some of this? In a world where sadness has been described as an epidemic and where mental health problems, such as anxiety and depression, affect up to one in four people, (308, 309) can eating plants really make us happier?

THE HAPPINESS EFFECT

In 2007 the 'fourth largest automobile insurance company in the United States' decided to find out if eating plants could make their employees happier. Doctors, dietitians and chefs visited the offices of the Government Employees Insurance Company once a week to educate their employees on how to make the switch to a plant-based diet. Lentil soup, rice and beans, minestrone, veggie burgers and bean burritos were all on the menu. The result? 'A significant increase in physical functioning, general health, vitality, and mental health over the 22-week study period.' Their employees became happier! One-third of participants reported better energy, and a quarter reported better sleep. The insurance company was happier too, as the staff who'd taken part in the programme became more productive in the workplace. (310)

This happiness effect has been observed in multiple studies. In 2018 the *British Medical Journal* published a review of the effects of a plant-based diet in the treatment of type 2 diabetes. Having analysed multiple studies conducted in the USA, Europe, New Zealand and Asia, they reported that alongside better blood sugar control and fewer overall symptoms of diabetes, patients who switched to a plant-based diet experienced 'significantly improved psychological well-being and quality of life'. (311)

If healthier food choices can improve our mood and feelings of well-being, what benefits might they have for people diagnosed with a serious mental health condition? In 2017 Australian psychiatrists recruited 67 adult volunteers with a formal diagnosis of clinical depression. Half the volunteers entered a programme of intensive social and emotional support. The other half took part in a healthy eating course. Their new meal plans were built around a traditional Mediterranean diet, emphasising daily intake of wholegrains, fruits, vegetables, nuts and legumes. After 12 weeks 32% of the healthy eating group had successfully improved their depressive symptoms, compared to just 8% of those who'd received social support alone. When it comes to depression, the psychiatrists concluded that improving a patient's diet could provide an effective treatment strategy. (312)

Personally, I've always found that taking time out to prepare and serve meals using the healthiest of ingredients helps me to relax and unwind. After a particularly demanding shift at the hospital, I can usually be found in the kitchen. Chopping vegetables is a wonderful antidote to a stressful day. A plant-based diet has so many overall benefits, it's difficult to tease out whether an improved mood is cause or effect. Weight loss, reduced cholesterol and improved digestive health could just make people feel happier. However, there are good biological reasons why people might experience increased feelings of well-being. Cutting out meat, poultry and fish significantly reduces your intake of arachidonic acid and advanced glycosylation end products, two substances that are thought to impact negatively on mood and brain health. (313, 314) Plant-based diets may also favourably affect the body's metabolism of tryptophan, a substance used by the brain to manufacture the 'happy hormone', serotonin. (315, 316) In older adults, higher levels of plant-derived nutrients, vitamins, antioxidants and folic acid in the bloodstream correlate with improved mood scores. (317-319)

The psychological benefits seem to increase with every portion of fruits and vegetables that you eat. Increasing to eight servings a day can have the same positive impact on mood and well-being as experienced when an unemployed person finds a new job. (320) In January 2020 a team of Polish researchers published a combined analysis of 61 studies covering tens of thousands of participants. (321) They found that a high total intake of fruits and vegetables is associated with higher levels of optimism and reduced psychological stress, and protects against depressive symptoms. It should come as no surprise that vegans report less stress and anxiety than omnivores. (322) On average, people who eat more plants really are happier.

YOUR GUT-BRAIN CONNECTION

To further understand exactly how eating plants might improve our mood, we first need to understand the 'microbiome-gut-brain axis'. This is an incredibly complex system that allows our microbes, our digestive system and our brain to communicate with each other. Those butterflies in your tummy before an important exam, and the gut feeling that tells you a risky new venture is going to be a success, these are both everyday examples of the microbiome-gut-brain axis at work. Our microbes, our gut and our brain are in constant communication. Information travels in both directions via nerves, hormones and other signalling mechanisms. (323)

The evidence that the gut and the microbiome might directly affect decision-making and mood is growing. Some researchers even believe that gut bugs can influence appetite and the foods we choose to eat! (324) In 2019 Austrian researchers showed that they could change volunteers' brain activity simply by asking them to drink a probiotic mix of gut-friendly bacteria for four weeks. (325) Another team showed that a probiotic bacteria supplement resulted in multiple benefits when given to adults with symptoms of stress. By supplementing their healthy gut microbes, volunteers experienced reduced symptoms of stress and anxiety, improved memory and cognition, enhanced serotonin activity, and lower levels of stress hormones. (326)

Changing your gut microbes may even improve the quality of your sleep. (327) Although the probiotic industry is excited at the potential of using their products to treat mood disorders, simply eating more plants to promote the growth of those healthy gut bacteria may be enough. Studies using various forms of fibre have shown promising results, including reductions in the stress hormone cortisol in healthy adults and improved anxiety scores in patients with irritable bowel syndrome. (328, 329)

A recent study revealed that people with adequate levels of certain bacteria may be more likely to have a better quality of life and less likely to suffer from depression. (329) The bacterial types that were linked to good mental health are called *Feacalibacterium* and *Coprococcus*. These two happen to be among the fibre-loving bacteria known to thrive on a plant-based diet. (331, 332) The main job of these bacteria is turning fibre into butyrate, one of the beneficial short-chain fatty acids that combat chronic inflammation in the gut and elsewhere. Multiple mechanisms have been proposed to explain exactly how this substance, produced by our gut microbiome when we eat plants, could protect our brain health. (333) While the science is in its infancy, it's fascinating to discover that the same fibre-loving gut microbes that maintain our physical health may play an equally important role in protecting our psychological well-being.

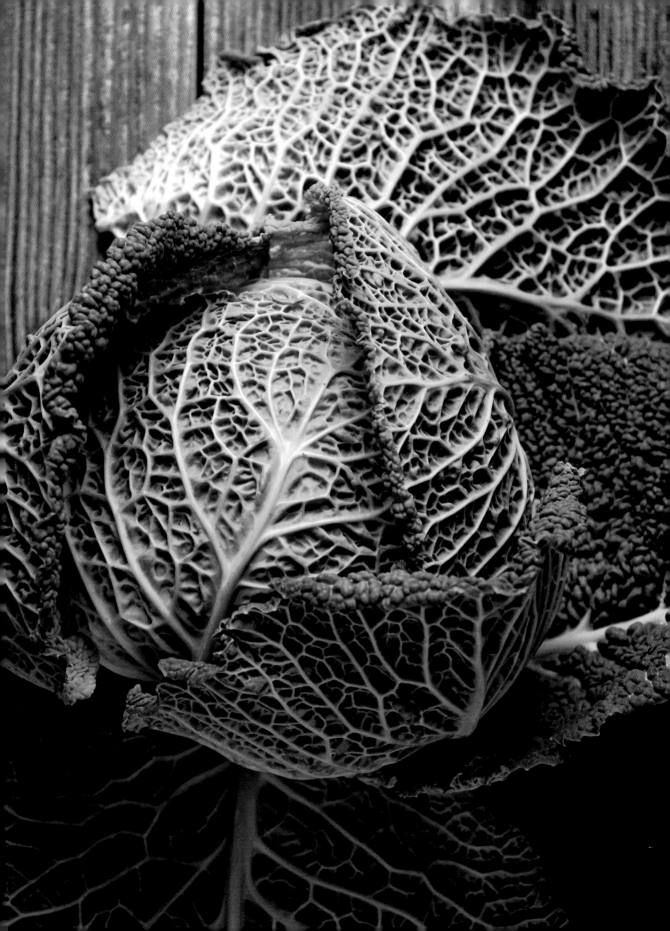

PROTECTING YOUR LONG-TERM BRAIN HEALTH

Alzheimer's disease is one of the most feared forms of dementia. Like many chronic illnesses, it is a disease that has become increasingly common in high-income countries, affecting 1 in 10 people over the age of 65. (334) Although there are genes that increase your risk of developing Alzheimer's disease, these account for less than 5% of cases. (335) In the United States, almost 500,000 people are diagnosed with Alzheimer's disease each year. (336)

But there is hope: a healthy lifestyle and diet can prevent the majority of cases. (337) It's never too early to start protecting your long-term brain health. The very earliest changes in memory and behaviour can start in your mid-thirties. (338) Not smoking, keeping your alcohol intake low, getting good-quality sleep and staying both physically and mentally active all help. And so does eating a plant-powered diet. (339)

Like all our organs, our brain depends on a constant supply of blood from our heart. In 'healthy heart' I described the many ways that a plant-based diet protects our blood vessels as we age. If the blood vessels that supply our brain become unhealthy and clogged up with cholesterol, they are simply unable to deliver enough oxygen and nutrients to keep it healthy. A reduced blood supply causes brain cells to die off, leading to reduced cognitive function and memory loss. This condition – called vascular dementia – accounts for 15% to 20% of dementia cases in North America and Europe and may also be a key player in the development of Alzheimer's disease. (340)

In 2015 researchers examined the ability of the food we eat to prevent dementia. They recruited more than 900 older adults and monitored their food choices and brain health for almost five years. The result? Eating a healthy plant-powered diet appeared to prevent brain ageing. The foods that were linked with preserved brain function included wholegrains, vegetables, berries, beans and nuts. (341) Participants who made the healthiest food choices maintained the mental agility of a person 7.5 years younger than them. These findings were not surprising; researchers had known for decades that even among populations that maintain a healthy diet and lifestyle, those who avoid consuming meat, poultry and fish entirely can cut their risk of developing dementia in half. (342) The same plant-powered meals that can combat chronic inflammation and improve your psychological well-being today will also help you to preserve your physical and cognitive health for decades to come. (343-352)

HOW HAS A PLANT-BASED DIET AFFECTED YOUR MOOD AND MENTAL HEALTH?

Here are some of the replies I received when I posed this important question to my followers on Instagram

'I feel more balanced. I feel more able to understand and influence my mood.' – Darren

'I feel like every meal is designed to nourish, not just fill, and that makes me feel so great.' – Brian

'I have much more energy and generally feel lighter both mentally and physically.' – Aisling

'Almost five years plant-based, I'm happier and healthier than ever. No regrets!' – Chris

'I'm less stressed and calmer, with reduced food anxiety.' – Gemma

'Happier, calmer with increased mental clarity.' – Charlotte

This was not a scientific survey by any means, but the answers are certainly in keeping with the science. A whole-food plant-based diet really can make you happier!

LESSONS FROM THE PANDEMIC

In early 2020 the novel coronavirus pandemic took hold and our world changed for ever. I soon found myself on the medical front line, treating hospitalised patients who'd been affected by COVID-19. Despite finding themselves seriously unwell with this new and poorly understood disease, and even with the added stress of being on an isolation ward where no visiting hours and staff clad in full PPE were the norm, many of our patients went out of their way to crack a joke or to share their gratitude. Even in such drastic circumstances, they did the best they could to cheer up the ward staff and keep us going. I was humbled by their bravery. Like all doctors and health professionals, I was also awestruck by just how quickly people could be overwhelmed by COVID-19. Patients who arrived on our unit looking quite well could be left struggling for their lives within hours. There were many heart breaking cases.

Early reports from China warned us that patients diagnosed with COVID-19 who already had high blood pressure, cardiovascular disease or type 2 diabetes were more likely to run a severe course, with increased risk of hospitalisation, ventilation, and death. (353) As the pandemic spread to the United States, a similar picture emerged. In March 2020, almost 90% of patients admitted to COVID-19 wards in New York state had more than one pre-existing chronic illness. (354)

Reports from around the globe have remained consistent. When the novel coronavirus seeks out a host to infect, it doesn't differentiate between young or old, healthy or frail, plant-based or omnivore. However, once the infection takes hold, your chances of fighting it successfully very much depend on your underlying health. Patients with high blood pressure, heart disease, type 2 diabetes, cancer or obesity are at a serious disadvantage in the fight to survive. (353-356)

We already knew that these chronic illnesses can steal years from our healthy life span. COVID-19 has placed a spotlight on just how vulnerable they can make us when our bodies are placed under extreme pressure. A recent study examining just how common these risk factors are in the US makes for sobering reading. Incredibly, 10.8% of US adults now live with type 2 diabetes and 8.5% have been diagnosed with heart disease. Overall, more than 1 in 5 employed US adults are now living with multiple chronic illnesses and 56% are at risk of hospitalisation with COVID-19 due to their poor underlying health. (357)

Experts have also pointed to the fact that, just like SARS and Swine flu, COVID-19 is a zoonotic disease – one caused by a virus that successfully leapt the species barrier from animals to humans. The animal-product-heavy Standard Western Diet has proven itself to be even more hazardous to human health than previously thought. The dietary habits that require us to raise more than 70 billion land animals per year for food – the majority of them kept in cramped and unsanitary conditions in close proximity to humans – make such cross-species leaps almost inevitable. (358, 359) In July 2020 the United Nations published a comprehensive report outlining the actions needed to prevent the next pandemic. That report described 'increasing human demand for animal protein' as the planet's number one driver of zoonotic diseases. (359)

It's difficult to feel optimistic in the era of coronavirus. But hidden among all this tragedy is a message of hope. Many of the underlying conditions that place us at risk of serious complications of this new infection can be prevented, halted, and even reversed by a healthy lifestyle and by a healthier approach to food. More people than ever now recognise the importance of plant-based food choices for both individual and global health.

As researchers work to develop a safe and effective vaccine, social distancing and the wearing of masks will remain vital to help curb the spread of the virus. But there is other important work to do. As individuals, governments, and health authorities seek assistance in protecting our health and preventing the next zoonotic pandemic, we each have an opportunity to make our voice heard. Food systems can change. We can drive that change. The plant-based diet revolution has never been more relevant or more urgent!

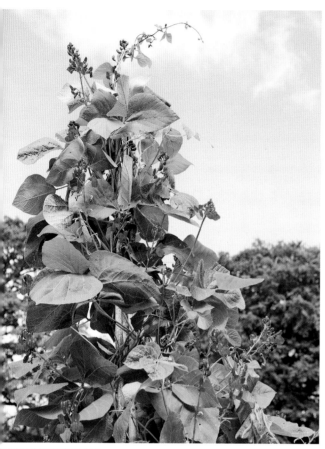
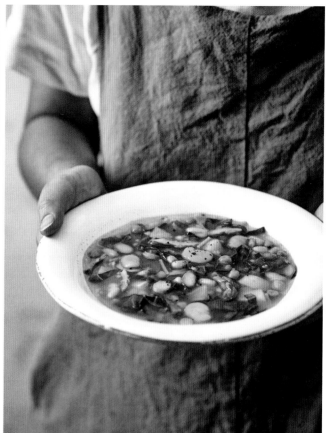
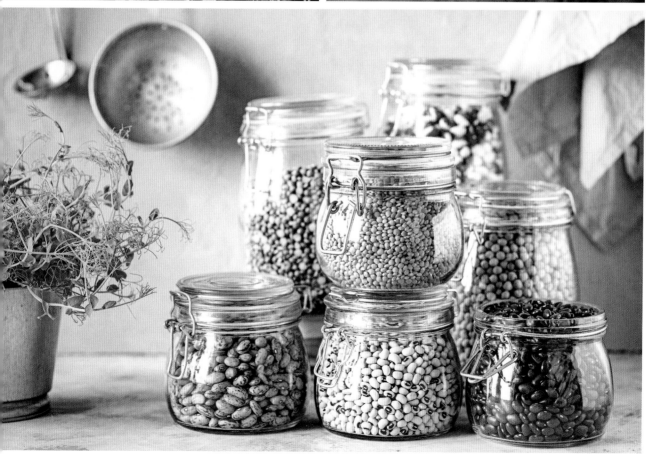

PART THREE

RECIPES FOR THE REVOLUTION

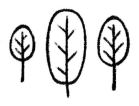

GETTING THE BASICS RIGHT

These recipes are built exclusively from plants. Fruits, vegetables, wholegrains, legumes, nuts, seeds, herbs and spices combined in delicious meals to fuel your microbiome and set you on the path to a healthier gut, heart, body and mind.

Alongside each recipe you'll find the following key information:

PLANT SCORE: The number of plants that the recipe puts on your plate. The key to achieving a healthy gut microbiome is increasing the total number of unique plants in your diet. Use this number to keep track of your weekly total. Hitting more than 30 different plants per week is a great initial target. Although herbs and spices also bring health benefits, the plant score only counts whole plants and ingredients that are used in significant quantities.

GRAMS OF FIBRE PER SERVING: The main meals contain an average 18g of fibre per serving, while the lighter meals have an average of 12g. The minimum recommended fibre intake for an adult is 30g per day. That number should really be regarded as a *minimum* rather than a target. By making these recipes a regular part of your day, you'll soon be eating as much fibre as the healthiest populations in the world.

GRAMS OF PROTEIN PER SERVING: Where do you get your protein? From plants! The total daily protein requirement for an average female is 45g, while the average male needs 55g. If you're an active person then your personal protein requirement is likely to be higher. Whatever your requirement, these recipes have got you covered. The main meals contain an average 24g of protein per serving, while the lighter meals have an average of 15g.

GLUTEN INFORMATION: The recipes for the revolution include plenty of gluten-free options that do not compromise on taste. We've also provided easy gluten-free swaps whenever possible. These are clearly marked on each recipe.

If you have specific caloric requirements or macronutrient needs, you can access the full calorie count and nutritional content for each recipe and the 28-Day Revolution meal plans at alandesmond.com/revolution

A QUICK GUIDE TO SALT, PEPPER & SEASONING

The seasoning of a dish is a very personal thing: one person's bland is another person's intense. Freshly ground black pepper gives a warm, gentle spicing and is often best added at the end of a dish. Salt acts like a volume switch that increases and amplifies flavours. Unfortunately, this means that salt is commonly used to make bland, unhealthy and processed foods taste better. It's easy to see why we have developed an increased tolerance for salt and therefore tend to season excessively. The more you cook from scratch, the more you'll control the seasoning of your food. A good rule is to taste and tweak as you go. Try using a flaky sea salt; it has a better flavour, you'll use less, and it contains no artificial additives or anti-caking agents. Over time you'll find that your use of salt will decrease to allow the herbs, spices and true flavours of the meal to shine through.

There are three flavourings naturally high in salt that are often used to add a deep, savoury note to your cooking.

MISO is a fermented rice or soybean paste with a deeply savoury flavour, often used to enrich broths, stews or dressings. White miso is light, almost 'summery', while brown miso has a deeper flavour and feels more 'wintry'. If any form of miso is used in a dish, you'll need little or no extra seasoning.

SOY SAUCE is made from fermented soybeans and, like tamari (its gluten-free counterpart, which tastes exactly the same), is high in sodium. When one or other of these sauces is used, you'll need little or no extra seasoning.

VEGETABLE STOCK can be bought in cube or powder form and will often have added salt to increase the savouriness, so be wary when salting dishes that include them. Try to buy stock cubes labelled 'low salt' and that are free from artificial additives and stabilisers. A quick homemade stock with no added salt is easily made: coarsely grate 1 large onion, 2 carrots and 2 celery sticks into 1 litre of water. Add 1 smashed garlic clove, 2 bay leaves, 8 black peppercorns and a small sprig of thyme. Bring to a simmer and cook gently for 20 minutes before straining through a fine sieve. This light veggie stock will keep in your fridge for 3-4 days in an airtight container.

ADDED OILS

Fruits, vegetables, beans, nuts, seeds and wholegrains all naturally contain healthy plant-based oils in varying amounts. There is no real need to add more oil to your food on a regular basis. Some of our recipes do include extra virgin olive oil as an option. Due to its high content of mono-unsaturated fatty acids and phenols, extra-virgin olive oil has been shown to reduce inflammation and help to prevent heart disease. (352-355) However, like all processed oils, it also contains a lot of calories. If using extra virgin olive oil in your cooking, aim to use less than two tablespoons per day and always regard it as an optional extra.

You can roast and fry with far less oil than you think (or even with none at all). An exceptionally light coating is all that's really needed, so take the time to turn and thoroughly coat the veg in minimal oil rather than simply pouring oil all over it. When roasting without oil, use a non-stick tray or line it with baking parchment to avoid food sticking. A dash of stock or water can be added to prevent it scorching or drying, but be light-handed, or the food will steam and fail to take on some colour in the oven. Check on the veg regularly, as there's a fine line between golden and burnt.

FIVE TIPS FOR FRYING WITHOUT OIL

1 Start with a good-quality non-stick pan.

2 Allow the pan a few minutes to get nice and hot before you add the food.

3 Keep the food moving in the pan for a few minutes to allow the surface to caramelise and brown.

4 As the pan becomes dry, add a good splash of water or vegetable stock to deglaze the pan and prevent burning. The deglazed bits also add flavour.

5 Keep a close eye on the pan and turn or stir the food regularly. The liquid will eventually evaporate, so add a little more if additional cooking time is needed.

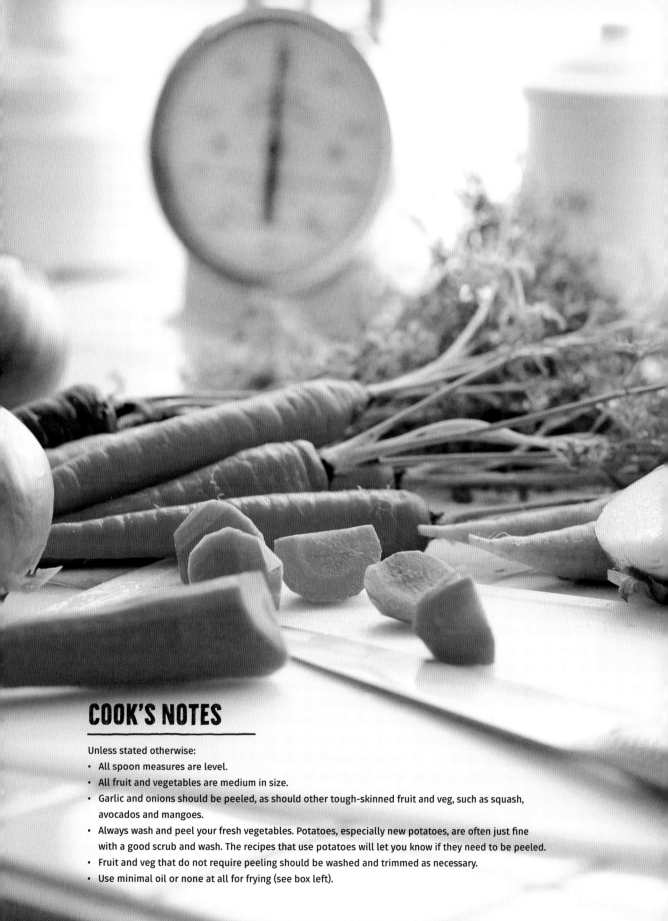

COOK'S NOTES

Unless stated otherwise:

- All spoon measures are level.
- All fruit and vegetables are medium in size.
- Garlic and onions should be peeled, as should other tough-skinned fruit and veg, such as squash, avocados and mangoes.
- Always wash and peel your fresh vegetables. Potatoes, especially new potatoes, are often just fine with a good scrub and wash. The recipes that use potatoes will let you know if they need to be peeled.
- Fruit and veg that do not require peeling should be washed and trimmed as necessary.
- Use minimal oil or none at all for frying (see box left).

BREAKFASTS

Perfect bowls of porridge 64

Simple cooked fruits and compotes 68

Easy wholegrain breads 70

Nut butter & banana on toast 72

Breakfast oat smoothies 74

Spring tofu hash 76

Spicy baked beans & sweet potato farls 78

Quick banana & blueberry pancakes 80

Spelt & buckwheat pancakes 80

Baked kedgeree with roast tomatoes, mushrooms & spinach 82

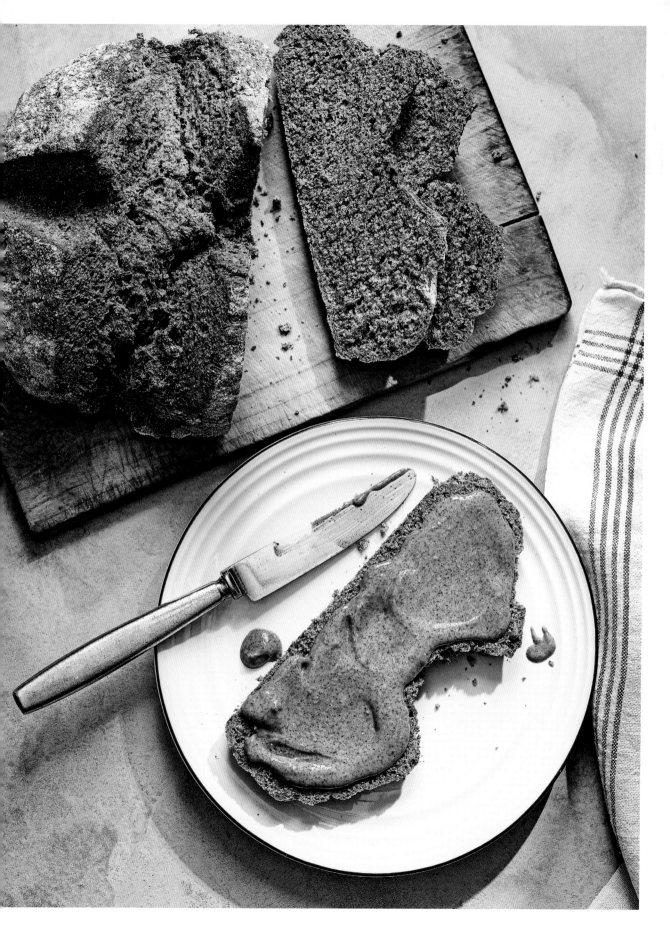

PERFECT BOWLS OF PORRIDGE

Porridge is the ultimate comfort breakfast. In cold weather I enjoy a bowl most mornings and love to mix it up between oats and other wholegrain options. They can take a little longer to prepare than simple oat porridge, but they are equally hearty and comforting.

SIMPLE OAT PORRIDGE

Serves 2 • Prep & cook: 20 minutes

PLANT SCORE: 1
FIBRE PER SERVING: 3.1g
PROTEIN PER SERVING: 5.2g
GLUTEN-FREE: YES, IF USING GLUTEN-FREE OATS

80g (1 cup) porridge oats

350ml (1½ cups) rice milk, or your favourite plant-based milk

1. Put the oats and milk in a pan over a medium heat and stir regularly as it cooks for 10–15 minutes. Add extra milk if the porridge is too thick for your liking.

2. Enjoy it plain or with a handful of berries, some plant-based yogurt, stewed apple, or any of the cooked fruits on pages 68–9. I like to top mine with a tablespoon of ground flaxseeds, a chopped banana and a teaspoon of peanut butter.

Variation
Use water instead of a plant-based milk, adding two chopped dates to the mixture to make the final porridge a little bit sweeter and creamier.

QUINOA PORRIDGE WITH BLACKBERRIES & PISTACHIOS

Instead of using the ingredient weights specified below, you can use volume measures when cooking quinoa. The rule is one part quinoa to two parts liquid. Always rinse your quinoa first or it can end up tasting bitter.

Serves 2 • Prep & cook: 25 minutes

PLANT SCORE: 3
FIBRE PER SERVING: 8g
PROTEIN PER SERVING: 13g
GLUTEN-FREE: YES

80g (1 cup) quinoa

350ml (1½ cups) plant-based milk, plus extra to finish

Dash of vanilla extract

1 tbsp maple syrup, or to taste

100g (⅔ cup) blackberries, fresh or defrosted

20g (scant ¼ cup) unsalted pistachios, roughly chopped

1. Rinse the quinoa thoroughly in a sieve under cold running water. Transfer to a saucepan on a moderate heat and cook gently for 3–4 minutes, until it smells toasty and has started to colour lightly. Take care not to burn it.

2. Add the milk, vanilla and maple syrup. Bring to a gentle simmer and cook for about 10 minutes, before adding half the blackberries. Cook for a further 6–8 minutes, or until soft and unctuous, adding a dash of water if it seems a little too dry.

3. Taste and tweak the sweetness to your liking. Serve topped with the remaining blackberries and a scattering of pistachios.

RYE BREAD PORRIDGE WITH ORANGE & PRUNES

Based on a traditional Danish dish that uses dark beer as the cooking liquid, this version uses plant milk instead. It's a lovely comforting porridge, ideal for a cold winter morning.

Serves 2 • Prep & cook: 15 minutes plus soaking time

PLANT SCORE: 3
FIBRE PER SERVING: 5.1g
PROTEIN PER SERVING: 8.9g
GLUTEN-FREE: NO

150g (5oz) stale rye bread

300ml (1¼ cups) almond or oat milk

Zest and juice of 1 small orange

2 tbsp water

4 pitted prunes

1 tbsp maple syrup, or to taste

¼ tsp ground cinnamon, or to taste

1. Crumble the rye bread into a food processor or blender and blitz it into coarse breadcrumbs. Place them in a large saucepan and add the milk. Leave to soak for at least 30 minutes, or preferably overnight.

2. In the meantime, tip the orange juice and water into a small saucepan. Add the prunes and bring to a simmer for 5 minutes. Set aside to plump up and soften. (This can be done the night before if soaking the bread overnight.)

3. When you are ready to cook the porridge, place the pan of bread on a gentle heat and stir in the maple syrup and cinnamon. Simmer for 10 minutes, stirring continuously, until you have a smooth porridge. For an even smoother texture, you can finish it with a hand blender. Thin with a dash of hot water if it feels too thick.

4. Taste and adjust the sweetness and cinnamon to your liking. Serve immediately topped with the soaked prunes and orangey syrup. Garnish with the orange zest to make this porridge even fancier.

BROWN RICE PORRIDGE WITH COCONUT, CASHEW & MANGO

Any leftovers of this delicious mixture can be stored in the fridge and later served as a dessert with some warm stewed fruit and a grating of dark chocolate.

Serves 2 • Prep & cook: 45 minutes plus overnight soak

PLANT SCORE: 4
FIBRE PER SERVING: 5.9g
PROTEIN PER SERVING: 8.4g
GLUTEN-FREE: YES

90g (½ cup) brown basmati rice

40g (1½ oz) unsalted cashew nuts

350ml (1½ cups) boiling water

¼ tsp ground cardamom

500ml (2 cups) coconut milk (drinking variety, not canned type)

1 tbsp maple syrup, or to taste

1 small mango, peeled, stoned and diced

1½ tbsp toasted coconut flakes

1. Place the rice and cashews in separate bowls of cold water and leave to soak overnight.

2. Drain the rice and place it in a large saucepan with the boiling water and cardamom. Bring to a simmer and cook for 25 minutes, until the rice is just tender.

3. Meanwhile, drain and rinse the cashews. Place them in a food processor or blender with the coconut milk and maple syrup. Blend until smooth.

4. Tip the blended milk into the rice and cook for a further 15–20 minutes, until soft and porridge-like. Taste and tweak the sweetness to your liking.

5. Serve topped with the fresh mango and a scattering of toasted coconut flakes.

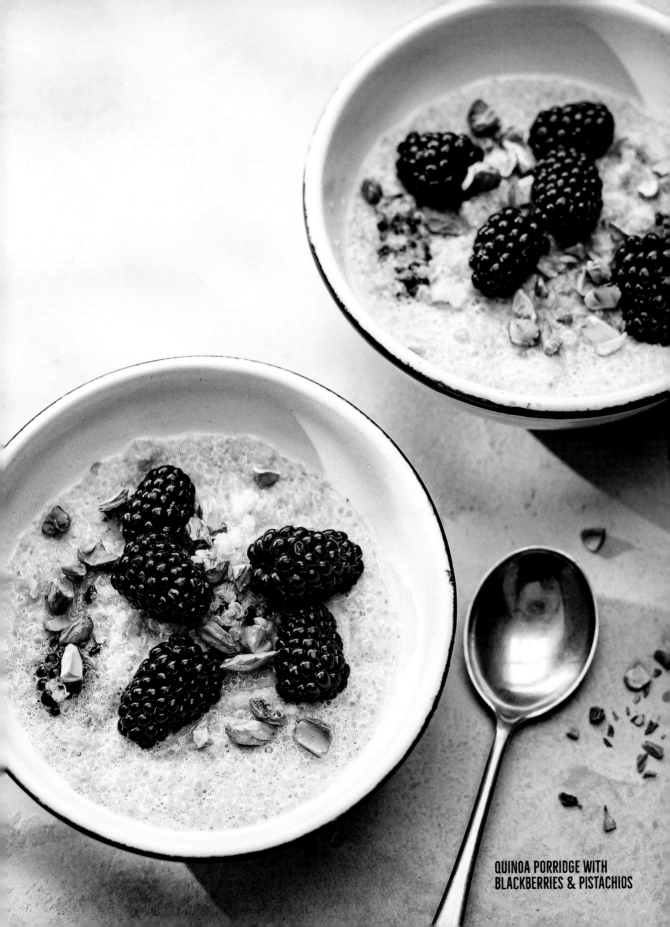

QUINOA PORRIDGE WITH
BLACKBERRIES & PISTACHIOS

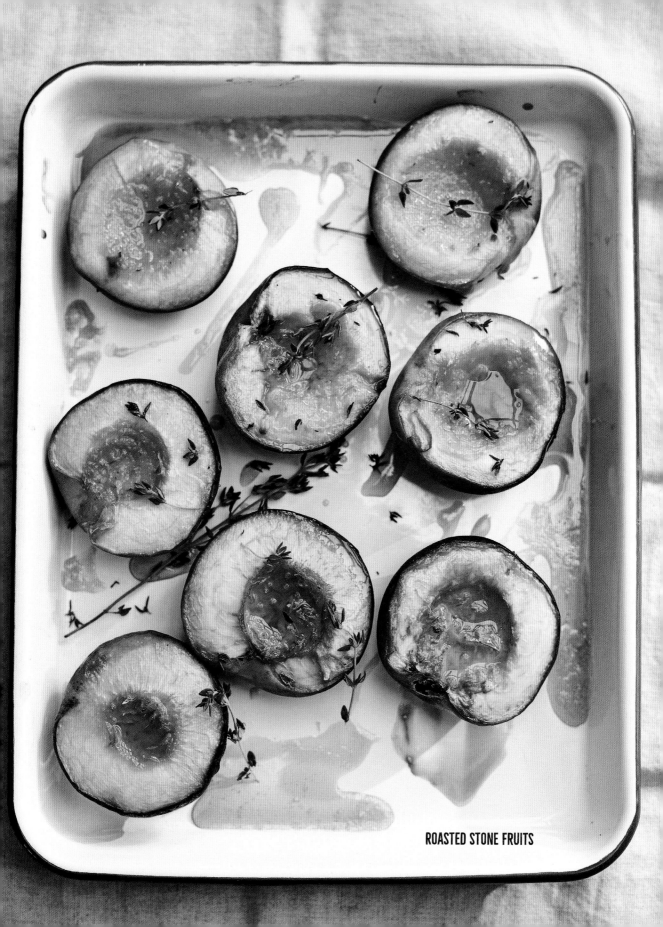

ROASTED STONE FRUITS

SIMPLE COOKED FRUITS & COMPOTES

These lightly sweetened compotes go perfectly with pancakes, wholemeal bread, toast or porridge. They don't take long to make and are definitely worth the effort. They'll keep in an airtight container in the fridge for 2–3 days.

Each recipe makes 2 servings

SPICED PLUMS

Prep & cook: 25 minutes

PLANT SCORE: 2
FIBRE PER SERVING: 2.3g
PROTEIN PER SERVING: 0.6g
GLUTEN-FREE: YES

5 plums, halved and stoned

1 small cinnamon stick

1 star anise

Freshly grated nutmeg

1 tbsp maple syrup

Zest and juice of ½ orange

1. Preheat the oven to 200°C/Fan 180°C/400°F/Gas 6.

2. Place the plums in a snug-fitting roasting tin. Throw in the cinnamon stick, star anise and a cautious grating of nutmeg. Add the maple syrup, orange zest and juice, then stir to combine.

3. Bake for 20 minutes, or until soft and sweet.

ROASTED STONE FRUITS

Prep & cook: 25 minutes

PLANT SCORE: 1
FIBRE PER SERVING: 2.6g
PROTEIN PER SERVING: 1.1g
GLUTEN-FREE: YES

2 peaches or nectarines, or 4 apricots, halved and stoned

1 tbsp maple syrup

2 sprigs of thyme (optional)

1. Preheat the oven to 200°C/Fan 180°C/400°F/Gas 6.

2. Place the fruit in a snug-fitting roasting tin. Add the maple syrup and mix together.

3. Bake for 20 minutes, or until soft and sweet.

RHUBARB OR GOOSEBERRY

Both these summer fruits have a mouth-puckering sourness that can be tempered with a bit of maple syrup. You can judge it for yourself, but take care not to lose all the sharpness, as that is part of the charm.

Prep & cook: 15 minutes

PLANT SCORE: 1
FIBRE PER SERVING: 1.4g
PROTEIN PER SERVING: 0.5g
GLUTEN-FREE: YES

120g (1 cup) diced rhubarb, or 150g (1 cup) topped and tailed gooseberries

1 tbsp maple syrup, or to taste

1 tbsp water

1. Put all the ingredients into a small saucepan and cook gently over a low heat for 10 minutes, until the fruit collapses.

2. Taste and add a little more maple syrup if it seems too sharp.

PEARS & GINGER

Prep & cook: 15 minutes

PLANT SCORE: 1
FIBRE PER SERVING: 4.5g
PROTEIN PER SERVING: 0.6g
GLUTEN-FREE: YES

2 pears, peeled, cored and cut into 1cm (½ inch) dice

1 tbsp maple syrup

½ tsp ground ginger

2 cardamom pods, split

1. Pop all the ingredients into a saucepan and cook gently over a low heat for 10 minutes, until the pears have softened. Set aside to cool.

SUMMER BERRIES

Prep & cook: 10 minutes

PLANT SCORE 1
FIBRE PER SERVING: 2.6g
PROTEIN PER SERVING: 0.9g
GLUTEN-FREE: YES

200g (1⅓ cups) blueberries, blackberries, raspberries or sliced strawberries

1 tbsp maple syrup

½ lime

1. Place the fruit in a small saucepan with the maple syrup and a dash of water. Cook over a gentle heat for 5 minutes, or until the fruit has collapsed and softened.

2. If you fancy a hint of sharpness, add a little squeeze of lime; this works particularly well with blueberries.

STEWED APPLES & CINNAMON

Prep & cook: 12 minutes

PLANT SCORE: 1
FIBRE PER SERVING: 1.6g
PROTEIN PER SERVING: 0.5g
GLUTEN-FREE: YES

1 large cooking apple, peeled, cored and diced

1 tbsp maple syrup

Ground cinnamon, to taste

1. Place the apple and maple syrup in a small saucepan and place over a gentle heat. Cook for 5–6 minutes, until the apples have softened and started to break down but still retain some texture.

2. Add a pinch or two of cinnamon to taste.

PINEAPPLE OR MANGO

This recipe relies on the heat of the pan to quickly caramelise the natural fruit sugars. It can be a bit fierce, fast and smoky, so it helps if you have a good extractor fan. The aim is not to cook the fruit, but to get a deeper flavour.

Prep & cook: 10 minutes

PLANT SCORE: 1
FIBRE PER SERVING: 3.3g
PROTEIN PER SERVING: 0.8g
GLUTEN-FREE: YES

1 mango, peeled, stoned and cut into 1cm (½ inch) dice

or

½ pineapple, peeled, cored and cut into 1cm (½ inch) dice

1. Put a dry non-stick frying pan on a high heat for a couple of minutes until it is very hot.

2. Add the fruit and cook for 1 minute or so, stirring a couple of times until it is nicely browned and caramelised.

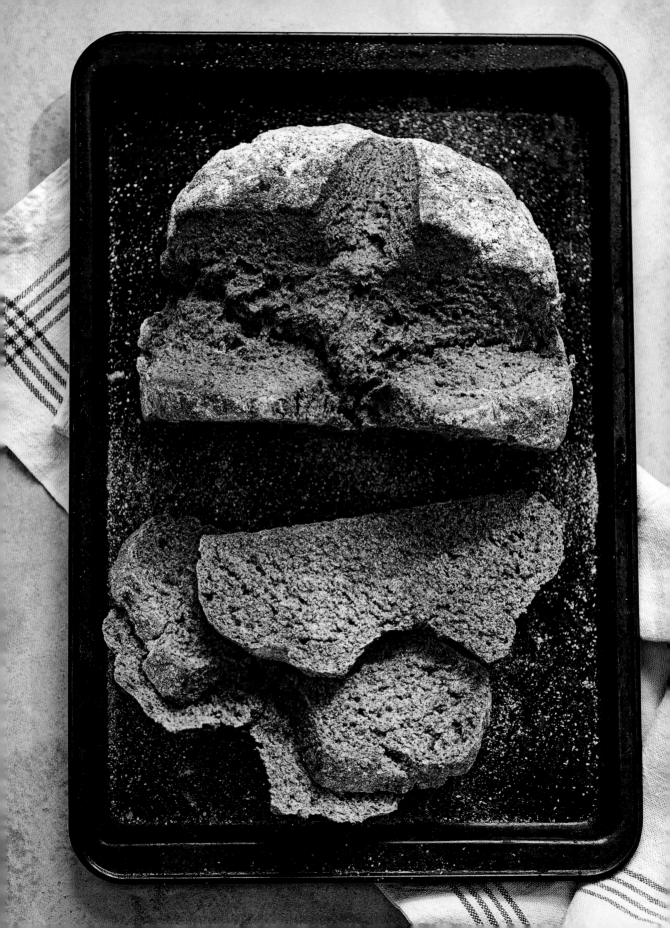

EASY WHOLEGRAIN BREADS

It's often difficult to find shop-bought breads without added sugars, emulsifiers or preservatives. Discover the simple joy of baking your own with these easy loaves. No lengthy kneading, rising or shaping required.

BROWN SODA BREAD

Based on a traditional Irish recipe, this brown bread is a perfect way to top up your daily intake of wholegrains. A slice will go nicely with any of the fruit compotes on pages 68-9, the Spicy baked beans on page 78 or any of the soups on pages 108–112.

Makes 1 loaf (8 slices or 4 servings)
Prep & cook: 45 minutes

PLANT SCORE: 3
FIBRE PER SERVING: 8.5g
PROTEIN PER SERVING: 13g (SAVOURY),
11g (SWEET)
GLUTEN-FREE: NO

1 tbsp ground flaxseeds (linseeds)

2 tbsp water

600g (4 cups) plain wholemeal flour, plus extra for dusting

2 tsp bicarbonate of soda

½ tsp sea salt

60g (scant ⅓ cup) pumpkin or sunflower seeds, for a savoury loaf (optional)

60g (⅓ cup) sultanas or chopped dates, for a sweeter loaf (optional)

400ml (1½ cups) plant-based milk

1 tbsp maple syrup

1 tbsp lemon juice

1. Preheat the oven to 200ºC/Fan 180ºC/400ºF/Gas 6. Mix the flaxseeds and water in a bowl and set aside to soak for at least 10 minutes.

2. Tip the flour and bicarbonate of soda and salt into a large bowl. Add the seeds or dried fruit, if using, and mix together with a spoon.

3. Add half the milk and continue to mix slowly. As the ingredients combine, add the soaked flaxseeds, maple syrup and lemon juice.

4. Finally, add the rest of the milk and bring it together into a dough – don't overmix or knead it or you'll affect the rise. Use your hands to shape it into a round loaf, adding a bit more flour if it is too wet and sticky.

5. Sprinkle some flour onto a non-stick baking tray. Place the loaf on it and score a deep cross in the top. Bake for 25–30 minutes, or until the loaf sounds hollow when tapped on the bottom. Leave to cool.

OAT BREAD

Another traditional Irish recipe, this bread is high in fibre and gluten-free. Try it with no-added-sugar jam or any of the cooked fruits on page 68, and a nice cup of tea.

Makes 1 loaf (8 slices or 4 servings)
Prep & cook: 1 hour 15 minutes

PLANT SCORE: 4
FIBRE PER SERVING: 4.2g
PROTEIN PER SERVING: 8.5g (SAVOURY);
6.7g (SWEET)
GLUTEN-FREE: YES, IF USING GLUTEN-FREE OATS

1 tbsp ground flaxseeds (linseeds)
2 tbsp water

400g (1¾ cups) natural soya yogurt

1 tbsp maple syrup

300g (3¾ cups) porridge oats

¼ tsp salt

2 tsp bicarbonate of soda

60g (scant ⅓ cup) pumpkin or sunflower seeds, for a savoury loaf (optional)

or

60g (⅓ cup) sultanas or chopped dates, for a sweeter loaf (optional)

1. Preheat the oven to 180ºC/Fan 160ºC/350ºF/Gas 4. Line a 1kg (2lb) loaf tin (about 20 x 12cm/8 x 5 inches) with non-stick baking paper.

2. Mix the ground flaxseeds and water in a large bowl and set aside to soak for at least 10 minutes. After that, stir in the yogurt and maple syrup.

3. Put the oats in a separate bowl and add the salt and bicarbonate of soda. If you wish, mix in the seeds or dried fruit. Once combined, add this dry mixture to the wet mixture and stir until you have a sticky dough. Place the dough in the prepared tin and bake for 1 hour. Set aside to cool.

NUT BUTTER & BANANA ON TOAST

This is a delicious combination. If you're in a hurry, just mash the bananas and spread them on the toasted rye bread, topping off with some nut butter. Unsweetened or 'natural' nut butters are widely available, but we've included a recipe to make your own.

HOMEMADE NUT BUTTER

I love homemade nut butters, which are free of the added sugars and oils often found in supermarket versions. Apart from a good food processor or blender, all you need is patience while you wait for the nuts to turn from a coarse, breadcrumb-like texture to a smooth paste as the oils are released. You can use the nuts raw, but toasting them first will give a deeper flavour.

Makes 1 x 300g (11oz) jar (10 servings)

PLANT SCORE: 2
FIBRE PER SERVING: 3.8g
PROTEIN PER SERVING: 5.9g
GLUTEN-FREE: YES

200g (1⅓ cups) whole almonds

100g (1 cup) walnut halves

Ground cinnamon

Sea salt

1. Preheat the oven to 180ºC/Fan 160ºC/350ºF/Gas 4. Lay the walnuts and almonds on a roasting tray and place in the oven for 4–5 minutes, until lightly coloured, and taking care not to burn them. Set aside to cool for 5 minutes.

2. Tip the nuts into a food processor or blender with a pinch of cinnamon and sea salt. Blitz them for 2 minutes, then scrape down sides with a spatula and blitz for another 2 minutes. Repeat this process of blitzing and scraping until the mixture becomes a paste. It may take a while, but will happen eventually.

3. When the texture is right, taste and adjust the seasoning to your liking.

Serves 2 • Prep & cook: 10 minutes

PLANT SCORE: 3
FIBRE PER SERVING: 11g
PROTEIN PER SERVING: 17g
GLUTEN-FREE: YES, IF USING GLUTEN-FREE BREAD

Extra virgin olive oil (optional)

2 firm bananas

4 slices dark, dense rye bread

80g (5 tbsp) nut butter (see box)

Raw cacao powder, for dusting

Maple syrup, to taste

1. Rub a large non-stick frying pan with a dash of oil (you won't need it if the non-stick surface is good) and put it over a medium heat.

2. Meanwhile, slice each unpeeled banana in half lengthways, then carefully remove the skin.

3. When the pan is hot, cook the bananas for 2–3 minutes on each side, until golden. Take care when flipping them because they soften as they cook. I use a spatula and a fork.

4. Lightly toast the bread and divide between 2 plates. Spoon some nut butter onto each slice and top with the caramelised banana. Dust with a little cacao powder, and a drizzle of maple syrup if you're feeling fancy.

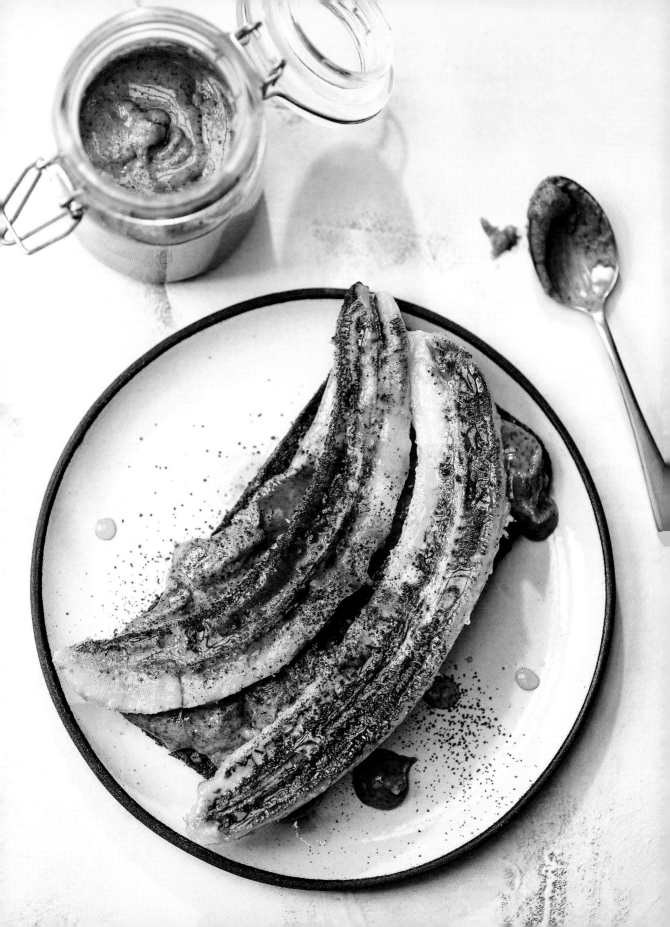

BREAKFAST OAT SMOOTHIES

Ideally we would always have time to sit and enjoy our breakfast. In the real world, we sometimes need to 'grab and go'. These oat-powered smoothies are deliciously filling and perfect for those busy mornings.

MOCHA OAT SMOOTHIE

Packed with protein, fibre, healthy fats and a caffeine hit, this breakfast-to-go is the ideal fuel for a busy morning. If you're sensitive to the jittery effects of caffeine, use a good-quality decaf coffee instead.

Serves 2 • Prep & cook: 10 minutes plus overnight soak

PLANT SCORE: 5
FIBRE PER SERVING: 7.4g
PROTEIN PER SERVING: 12g
GLUTEN-FREE: YES, IF USING GLUTEN-FREE OATS

50g (generous ½ cup) porridge oats
150ml (⅔ cup) black coffee
1–2 pitted dates
250ml (1 cup) almond milk
50g (scant ⅓ cup) cashew nuts
1 large ripe banana, chopped
1 tbsp raw cacao powder
Ground cinnamon
Maple syrup, to taste

1. Place the oats, coffee, dates and almond milk in a blender jug. Cover and leave in the fridge overnight.

2. Place the cashews in a bowl, cover with plenty of cold water and leave in the fridge overnight.

3. In the morning drain the cashews and add them to the blender along with the banana, cacao powder and a pinch of cinnamon. Blitz until smooth, adding more liquid if needed, and sweetening to taste with maple syrup.

4. Drink straight away, or pour into a flask to enjoy later. Leftovers will keep in the fridge to enjoy the next day.

BERRY OAT SMOOTHIE

You might be surprised to learn that this oat-and-berry-packed smoothie contains 7.5g of healthy plant-based protein to start your day.

Serves 2

PLANT SCORE: 5
FIBRE PER SERVING: 7.4g
PROTEIN PER SERVING: 7.5g
GLUTEN-FREE: YES, IF USING GLUTEN-FREE OATS

1 apple, coarsely grated
75g (1 cup) porridge oats
400ml (1¾ cups) oat milk
1 tbsp lemon juice
100g (⅔ cup) fresh or frozen mixed summer berries
Maple syrup, to taste (optional)

1. Combine the apple, oats and oat milk in a blender jug, then stir in the lemon juice. Cover and leave in the fridge overnight.

2. In the morning add the berries and blend until smooth. Add more oat milk if needed. Taste and add a little more sweetness if you like.

TROPICAL OAT SMOOTHIE

Mango, coconut and passionfruit make for a classic tropical combination. By adding the oats and some extra fruit you can enjoy a sunny breakfast-to-go whatever the weather.

Serves 2 • Prep & cook: 10 minutes plus overnight soak

PLANT SCORE: 5
FIBRE PER SERVING: 8.6g
PROTEIN PER SERVING: 5.9g
GLUTEN-FREE: YES, IF USING GLUTEN-FREE OATS

1 apple, coarsely grated

60g (¾ cup) porridge oats

400ml (1¾ cups) coconut milk (drinking variety rather than canned)

1 small banana

1 mango, peeled, stoned and sliced

1 passionfruit

1. Combine the apple, oats and coconut milk in a blender jug. Cover and leave in the fridge overnight.

2. In the morning add the banana, mango and passion fruit pulp. Blitz together until smooth, adding more milk if needed to give you a drinkable smoothie.

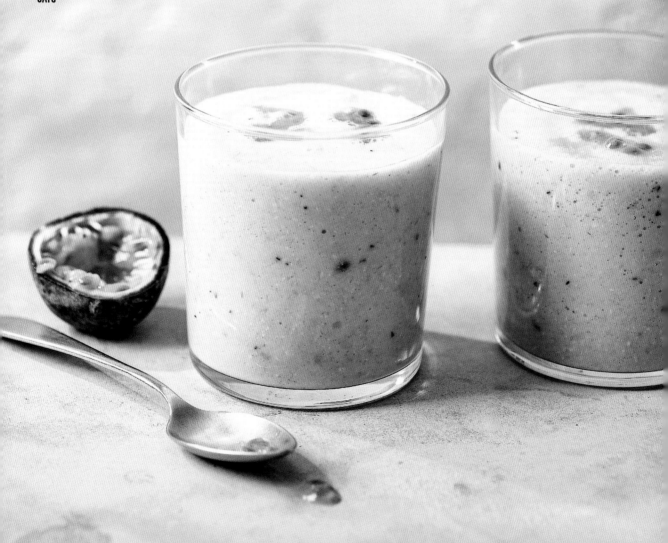

SPRING TOFU HASH

Tofu is an incredibly versatile and satisfying ingredient. You'll find it in quite a few of our recipes. Many supermarkets now stock silken, firm and extra firm varietes and brands that have been smoked, marinaded or pre-flavoured. A plain or smoked extra-firm tofu will work great in this savoury breakfast.

Serves 2
Prep & cook: 35 minutes

PLANT SCORE: 5
FIBRE PER SERVING: 9g
PROTEIN PER SERVING: 23g
GLUTEN-FREE: YES

400g (14oz) new potatoes, cut into 2cm (¾ inch) chunks and wedges

200g (7oz) firm or extra-firm tofu

¼ tsp ground turmeric

½ tsp ground cumin

½ tsp smoked paprika

2 tbsp extra virgin olive oil

4 radishes, cut into wedges

150g (5oz) asparagus, trimmed and cut into 2cm (¾ inch) pieces

3 spring onions, thinly sliced

1 lemon, cut into wedges

Small handful of fresh parsley, finely chopped

Sea salt and freshly ground black pepper

1. Place the potatoes in a saucepan, cover with cold water and bring to the boil. Simmer for 8–10 minutes, or until very nearly cooked. Drain when ready.

2. Meanwhile, drain the tofu, place it in a bowl and use a fork to break it into coarse chunks. Stir in the turmeric, cumin and paprika. Set aside.

3. Heat the oil in a large frying pan. Add the potatoes and season lightly with salt and pepper. Sauté over a medium heat for 10 minutes, until they start to colour. Add the radishes and cook for 3 more minutes. Throw in the asparagus and spring onions and cook for a final 3–4 minutes, until everything is cooked through. Transfer to a plate and set aside.

4. Put the frying pan back on the heat and add the tofu mixture. Cook on a high heat for 2–3 minutes, until hot, adding a dash of water if it looks like catching in the pan.

5. Tip the reserved veg into the tofu pan, add a squeeze of lemon juice and tumble everything together to heat through. Taste and tweak the seasoning to your liking.

6. Divide the hash between 2 plates and garnish with parsley. Serve with lemon wedges for squeezing over.

Oil-free:
To sauté the potatoes, start with a hot non-stick pan. Add the parboiled potatoes and keep them moving until they start to brown. Add 4 tablespoons water and simmer on a medium heat for 10 minutes. Stir occasionally and add an extra dash of water whenever the pan dries out.

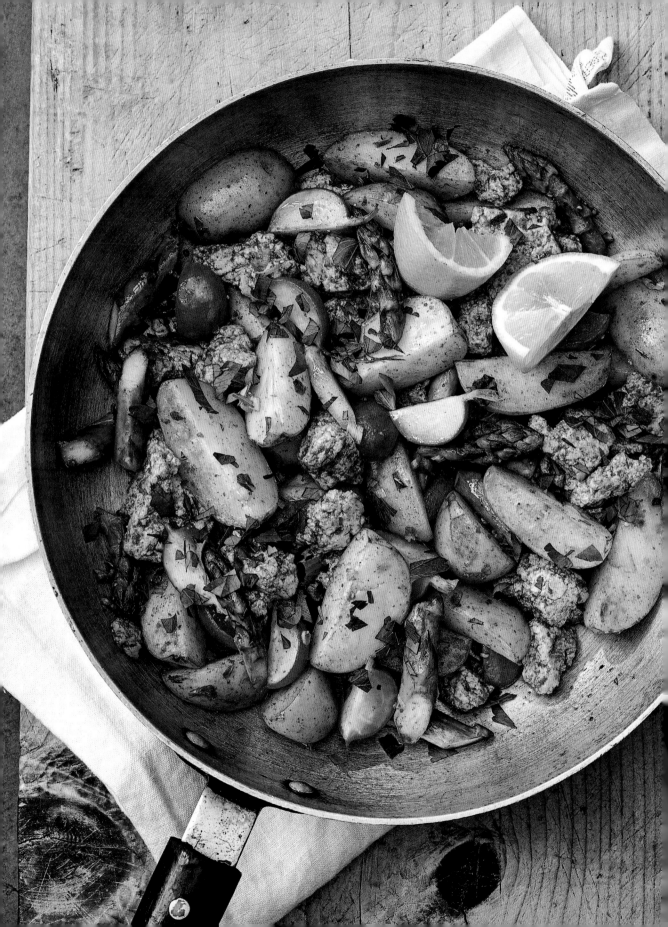

SPICY BAKED BEANS & SWEET POTATO FARLS

This recipe takes beans on toast to a whole new level. Try adding a little oregano or thyme to the farl dough for extra flavour. If you're gluten free, the beans can be made with tamari and will go great with a baked sweet potato (see page 86) or a lightly toasted slice of Oat bread (see page 71).

Serves 2
Prep and cook 35 minutes

PLANT SCORE: 7
FIBRE PER SERVING: 16g
PROTEIN PER SERVING: 17g
GLUTEN-FREE: THE FARLS: NO; THE BEANS: YES, IF YOU USE TAMARI RATHER THAN SOY SAUCE

1 red onion, sliced

Extra virgin olive oil (optional)

1 garlic clove, finely chopped

1 x 400g (14oz) can haricot beans, drained and rinsed

300g (1¼ cups) passata

1 tbsp harissa, or to taste (optional)

1 tbsp balsamic vinegar

1 tbsp tamari or soy sauce

Sea salt and freshly ground black pepper

Small handful of fresh parsley, freshly chopped, to garnish

FOR THE FARLS

300g (2 cups) sweet potatoes, peeled and diced

50g (⅓ cup) wholemeal flour

Extra virgin olive oil (optional)

1. Place the sweet potato for the farls in a saucepan of cold water and bring to the boil. Simmer until completely tender, about 15 minutes or so, then drain.

2. Meanwhile, put the onion in a large saucepan with ½ tablespoon olive oil (if using) or water and fry for 10 minutes, until soft and starting to caramelise. If they look like catching or burning, add an extra dash of water every so often to help them along.

3. Add the garlic to the onions and cook for 2 more minutes, then tip in the beans, passata, harissa (if using), vinegar and tamari. Season lightly with salt and pepper. Bring to a simmer and cook gently for 15 minutes, until the sauce is rich and thick.

4. While the beans cook, roughly mash the sweet potatoes and season lightly with salt and pepper. Fold in the flour until the mixture forms a rough dough; you might need to add a little more flour if it feels a bit sticky.

5. Put a non-stick frying pan over a medium heat. A rub of olive oil will help to prevent sticking. Put the dough into the pan and press it into a flat circle about 5mm (¼ inch) thick. Use a spatula to divide it into quarters. Cook for 4–5 minutes on each side, until nicely coloured and piping hot.

6. Taste the beans and tweak the harissa (if used) to your liking. If you want a thicker texture, whizz a quarter of the beans in a blender until smooth, then mix them back into the pan.

7. Serve each person 2 farls, generously topped with the beans and a scattering of parsley to finish.

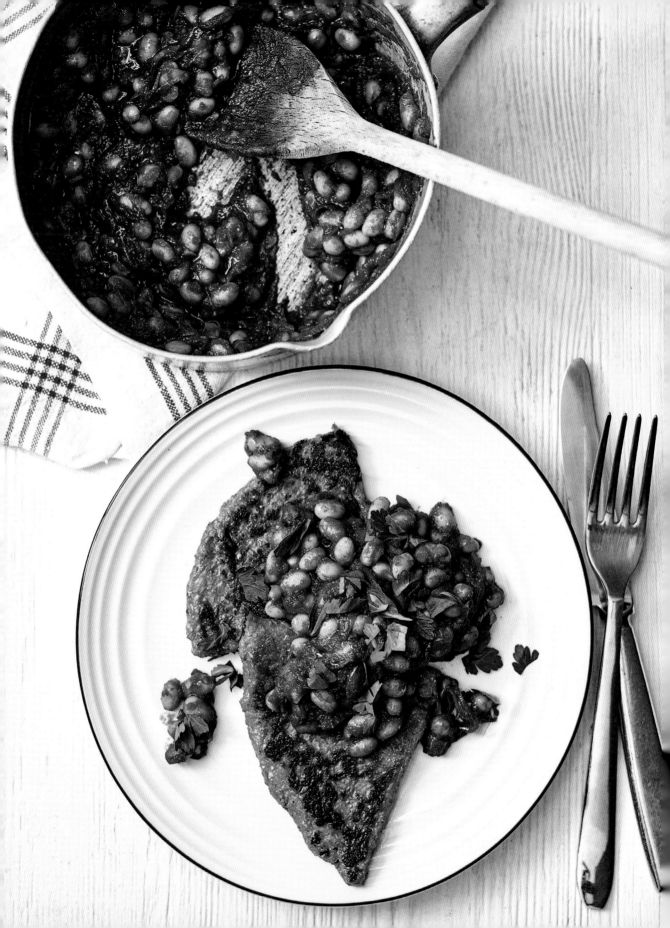

QUICK BANANA & BLUEBERRY PANCAKES

These American-style pancakes are a regular at our house. If you don't use all the batter, it will keep in the fridge overnight. Just add an extra splash of oat milk and give it a good stir before using.

Makes 8 small pancakes
Prep & cook: 20 minutes

PLANT SCORE: 4
FIBRE PER SERVING: 5.9g
PROTEIN PER SERVING: 1.8g
GLUTEN-FREE: NO

250ml (1 cup) oat milk or other plant milk

1 ripe banana

120g (¾ cup) wholemeal flour

1 tsp baking powder

1 tbsp peanut butter

Olive oil, for frying (optional)

150g (¾ cup) blueberries

Maple syrup, to drizzle

1. Place the milk, banana, flour, baking powder and peanut butter in a food processor or blender and whizz together until there are no floury lumps.

2. Heat a non-stick frying pan. A rub of oil will help prevent sticking. Put 3 or 4 separate dollops of batter in the pan, depending how much room there is. Sprinkle some blueberries onto each one, then cook over a medium heat until you see little bubbles appearing across the surface. Flip them over and cook the other side for a couple of minutes until golden brown and cooked through.

3. Serve the pancakes as you go, or keep a stack warm in a hot oven. Offer them with any leftover blueberries and a drizzle of maple syrup.

SPELT & BUCKWHEAT PANCAKES

The secret to making these wholegrain pancakes light and fluffy is to avoid overmixing the batter.

Makes 8
Prep & cook: 20 minutes

PLANT SCORE: 2
FIBRE PER SERVING: 2g
PROTEIN PER SERVING: 2.8g
GLUTEN-FREE: NO

75g (½ cup) wholemeal spelt flour

75g (scant ⅔ cup) buckwheat flour

1½ tsp baking powder

200ml (⅔ cup) almond or other plant milk

1½ tsp cider vinegar

1 tbsp maple syrup, or to taste

Extra virgin olive oil, for frying (optional)

1. Sift the flours and baking powder into a large bowl. In a separate bowl whisk the plant milk, vinegar and maple syrup together. Pour this into the dry ingredients and mix with a spatula just until the batter comes together with no floury lumps; don't overmix. Set aside for 10 minutes.

2. Heat a non-stick frying pan. A rub of oil will help prevent sticking. Put 3 or 4 separate dollops of batter in the pan, depending how much room there is, and cook the pancakes over a medium heat, until golden brown on the bottom. Flip over and cook the other side. Transfer to a plate and keep warm in a low oven while you cook the remainder. You should get about 8 pancakes.

3. Serve warm, topped with your favourite plant-based yogurt and a dollop of fruit compote (see pages 68–9).

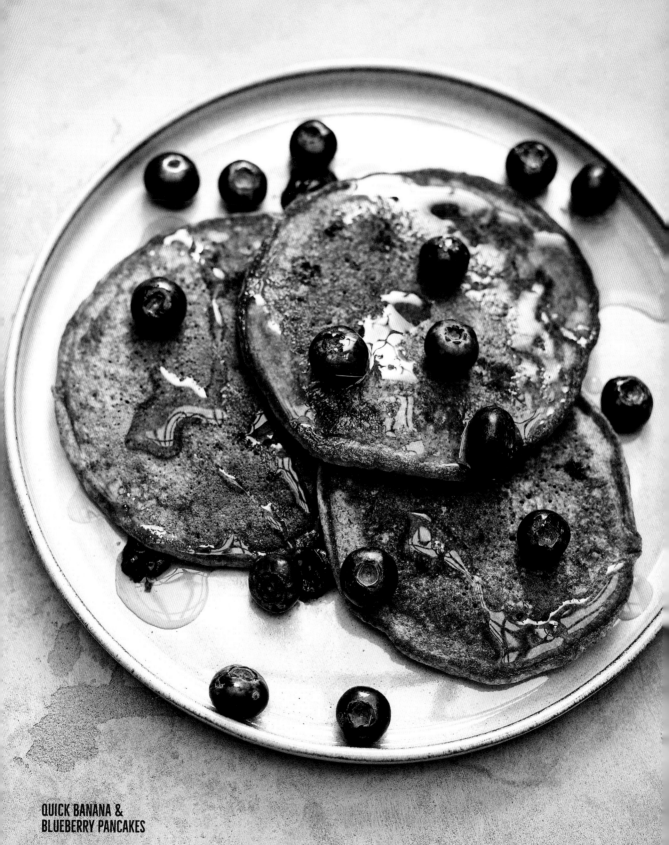

QUICK BANANA &
BLUEBERRY PANCAKES

BAKED KEDGEREE WITH ROAST TOMATOES, MUSHROOMS & SPINACH

Kedgeree is a breakfast favourite that originated from khichiri, a concoction of spiced lentils, rice, fried onions and ginger which dates back to 14th-century India. This recipe brings kedgeree a little bit closer to its plant-based roots. Add in a chilli or two to start your day with extra heat.

Serves 2
Prep & cook: 40 minutes

PLANT SCORE: 7
FIBRE PER SERVING: 13g
PROTEIN PER SERVING: 15g
GLUTEN-FREE: YES

4 Portobello mushrooms, stalks separated

2 large tomatoes, halved horizontally

Extra virgin olive oil, to drizzle

200g (1 generous cup) brown basmati rice, rinsed

2 spring onions, thinly sliced

1 tbsp medium-hot curry powder

6 cardamom pods, split open

1 teaspoon sweet smoked paprika

600ml (2½ cups) hot vegetable stock

100g (1 cup) baby spinach

1 tbsp dried seaweed flakes or crumbled nori sheets

Small handful of fresh parsley, roughly chopped

1 lemon, cut into fat wedges

Sea salt and freshly ground black pepper

1. Preheat the oven to 200°C/Fan 180°C/400°F/Gas 6.

2. Place the mushroom caps in a roasting tray, gill side up. Roughly chop the stalks and sit them back inside the caps. Sit a tomato half in the middle of each mushroom, drizzle over a little olive oil and season lightly. Add a dash of water to the tray to prevent the mushrooms scorching, then transfer to the oven. Bake for 25–30 minutes, or until the mushrooms are cooked through and the tomatoes are starting to colour and collapse.

3. Meanwhile, tip the rice into an ovenproof casserole dish or a saucepan. Add the spring onions, curry powder, cardamom pods, paprika and stock. Taste and season with a pinch of salt, if needed, and a few generous twists of black pepper. Mix well, pop on the lid and place it in the oven, on the shelf below the mushrooms, for 20–25 minutes, or until the rice is cooked. Alternatively, place the saucepan on the hob and cook over a gentle heat for 20 minutes, or until the rice Is cooked.

4. When the mushrooms come out of the oven, scatter the spinach into the tray and move it around for a minute or so, until it wilts from the heat.

5. To serve, stir the seaweed and half the chopped parsley into the rice and pile it onto your plates. Top each serving with some wilted spinach and 2 mushrooms. Garnish with the remaining parsley and some lemon wedges for squeezing over.

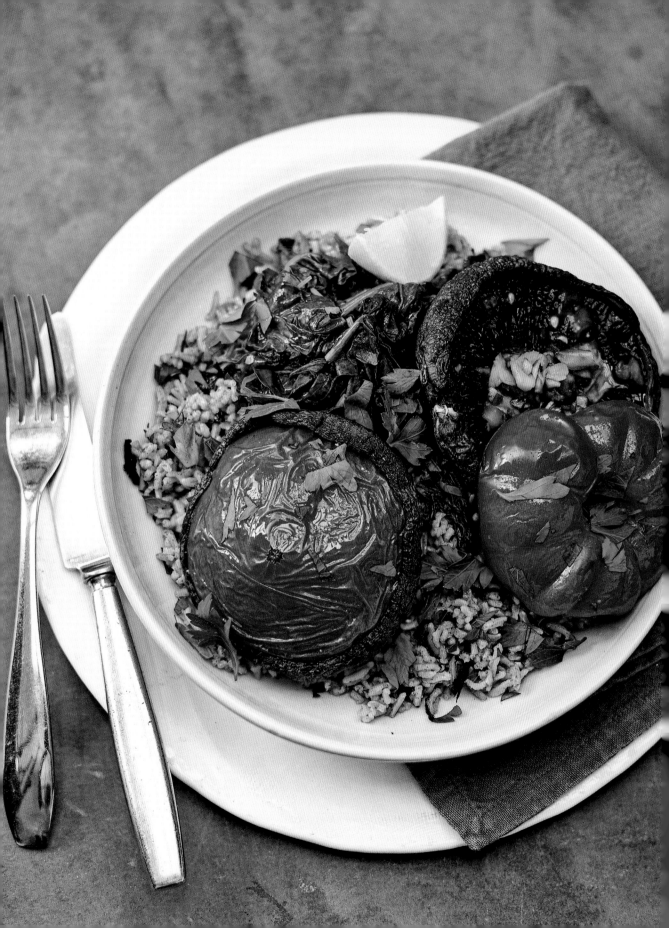

LIGHTER MEALS

Loaded sweet potatoes 86

Beyond hummus 90

Savoury farinata 92

Fiery noodle salad 96

MLT sandwich 98

Beetroot, sauerkraut & watercress sandwich 100

Spicy tofu rolls 102

Three fresh slaws 104

Speedy falafels and more 106

Chunky minestrone 108

Spanish red pepper soup 110

Spicy parsnip and lentil winter soup 112

Squash & raw kale quinoa salad 114

Wild rice super salad 116

Avocado on toast with four twists 118

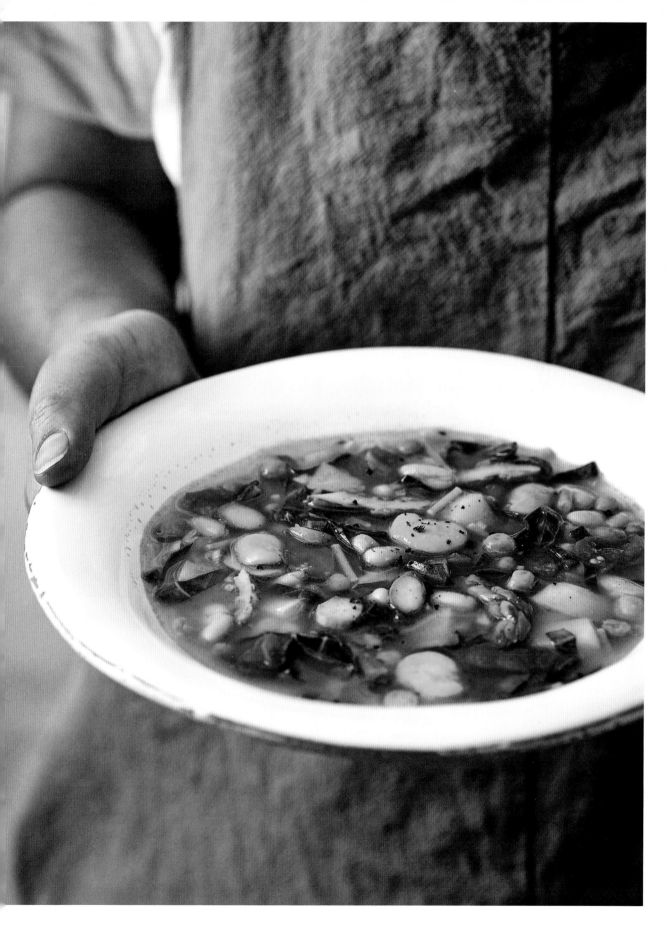

LOADED SWEET POTATOES

What could be easier than a simple baked potato topped with your favourite filling? Sweet potatoes have the advantage of baking a little bit faster than regular white potatoes, but both types of spud will work well with any of the fillings below.

BASIC BAKED SWEET POTATO

Serves 2 • Prep & cook: 1 hour

FIBRE PER SERVING: 3.9g
PROTEIN PER SERVING: 2g
GLUTEN-FREE: YES

2 large sweet potatoes

1. Preheat the oven to 200ºC/Fan 180ºC/400ºF/Gas 6.

2. Jab each sweet potato a few times with the tip of a knife. Place them directly on a shelf in the oven and bake for 45–60 minutes, until the centre is soft and the skin is crisp. Serve with your chosen topping, which can be made while the potatoes bake.

LOADED SWEET POTATO WITH SOUR CREAM & CHIVES

Don't be shy with the sour cream – it's made from tofu, so is extremely low in fat and packed with plant protein. Any leftover will keep in the fridge for 2–3 days; just stir it before serving.

Serves 2 • Prep & cook: 5 minutes

PLANT SCORE: 3
FIBRE PER SERVING: 11g
PROTEIN PER SERVING: 13g
GLUTEN-FREE: YES

2 sweet potatoes
1 x 300g (11oz) natural silken tofu
1 tbsp apple cider vinegar
Small handful of fresh chives, chopped (leek greens or wild garlic also work)

1. Bake the potatoes as described in Basic sweet potato recipe.

2. Meanwhile, place the tofu and vinegar in a blender and whizz until smooth. Spoon the mixture over your potato, sprinkle with the chives and serve.

LOADED SWEET POTATO WITH CHICKPEA TABBOULEH

The soft chickpeas contrast well with the crisp veg and fresh herbs. Don't be shy with the lemon juice – it brings the whole thing to life.

Serves 12 • Prep & cook: 15 minutes

PLANT SCORE: 7
FIBRE PER SERVING: 20g
PROTEIN PER SERVING: 17g
GLUTEN-FREE: YES

1 x 400g (14oz) can chickpeas, drained and rinsed
3 tomatoes, deseeded and finely diced
½ cucumber, deseeded and finely diced
½ small red onion, finely diced
Large handful of fresh parsley, finely chopped
8 large fresh mint leaves, finely chopped
Ground cinnamon
1 tbsp extra virgin olive oil (optional)
1 lemon

1. Bake the potatoes as described in Basic sweet potato recipe.

2. Meanwhile, roughly chop the chickpeas on a board until they are a similar size to your diced vegetables. Throw them into a bowl with the veg, herbs and a pinch of cinnamon. Add the oil (if using) and season to taste with pepper and salt. Finish with a generous squeeze of lemon.

LOADED SWEET POTATO WITH JERK BLACK BEANS & PEPPERS

Jerk seasoning, available from most supermarkets, is supposed to have a kick to it, but brands will differ in strength. If you like your food spicy, add an extra shake or two.

Serves 2 • Prep & cook: 40 minutes

PLANT SCORE: 7
FIBRE PER SERVING: 29g
PROTEIN PER SERVING: 23g
GLUTEN-FREE: YES

2 sweet potatoes

1 tbsp extra virgin olive oil (optional)

1 red onion, sliced

2 red peppers, deseeded and sliced

1½ tbsp jerk seasoning

1 x 400g (14oz) can black beans, drained and rinsed

1 x 400g (14oz) can chopped tomatoes

1 tbsp peanut butter

1 lime

Small handful of fresh coriander, chopped

Sea salt and freshly ground black pepper

1. Bake the potatoes as described in Basic sweet potato recipe.

2. Meanwhile, warm the olive oil (if using) or a few tablespoons water in a large saucepan. Add the onion and peppers and cook gently for 15 minutes, until softened. Add an extra dash of water if they look like catching at any point.

3. Throw in the jerk seasoning and cook for 1 minute, then add the beans, tomatoes and a half-can of water. Stir in the peanut butter. Taste and season to your liking with ground pepper and a pinch of sea salt. Cook for about 20 minutes, until it has thickened into a rich sauce. When ready, add a squeeze or two of lime.

4. Spoon a generous dollop of the beans into each sweet potato and sprinkle with the chopped coriander.

LOADED SWEET POTATO WITH SWEETCORN & CHARD

The smokiness of the paprika and the sharpness of the pickles combine to give this filling a real lift. If you can't find chard, use baby spinach, stalks and all, but stir it through just before serving.

Serves 2 • Prep & cook: 40 minutes

PLANT SCORE: 6
FIBRE PER SERVING: 11g
PROTEIN PER SERVING: 11g
GLUTEN-FREE: YES

2 sweet potatoes

150g (4 cups) chard

½ tbsp extra virgin olive oil (optional)

Sweetcorn kernels from 3 cobs, or about 300g (1¼ cups) canned sweetcorn

1 garlic clove, finely chopped

½ tsp dried thyme

½ tsp smoked paprika

300ml (1¼ cups) vegetable stock or water

2 spring onions, very finely sliced

2 tbsp chopped gherkins, or pickled jalapeños if you want some heat

1. Bake the potatoes as described in Basic sweet potato recipe.

2. Meanwhile, strip the chard leaves away from the stalks. Finely dice the stalks and roughly chop the leaves.

3. Warm ½ tablespoon olive oil or a few tablespoons water in a large saucepan. Cook the chard stalks gently on a low heat for 5 minutes, until softened. Add a dash of water if they look like catching.

4. Add the sweetcorn, garlic, thyme and paprika to the stalks and cook gently for another 5 minutes, stirring occasionally to make sure the paprika doesn't stick and burn. Add the stock and season lightly with salt and pepper. Simmer for 20 minutes, until the corn is tender and most of the liquid has disappeared.

5. Finally, stir in the chard leaves, spring onions and gherkins. Cook for 5 minutes to wilt the chard.

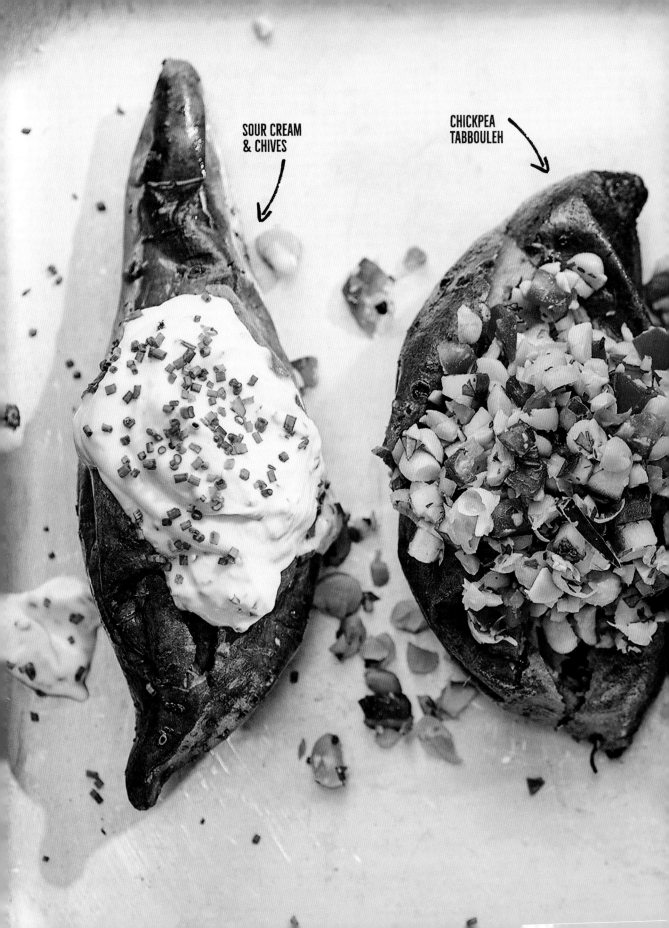

SOUR CREAM
& CHIVES

CHICKPEA
TABBOULEH

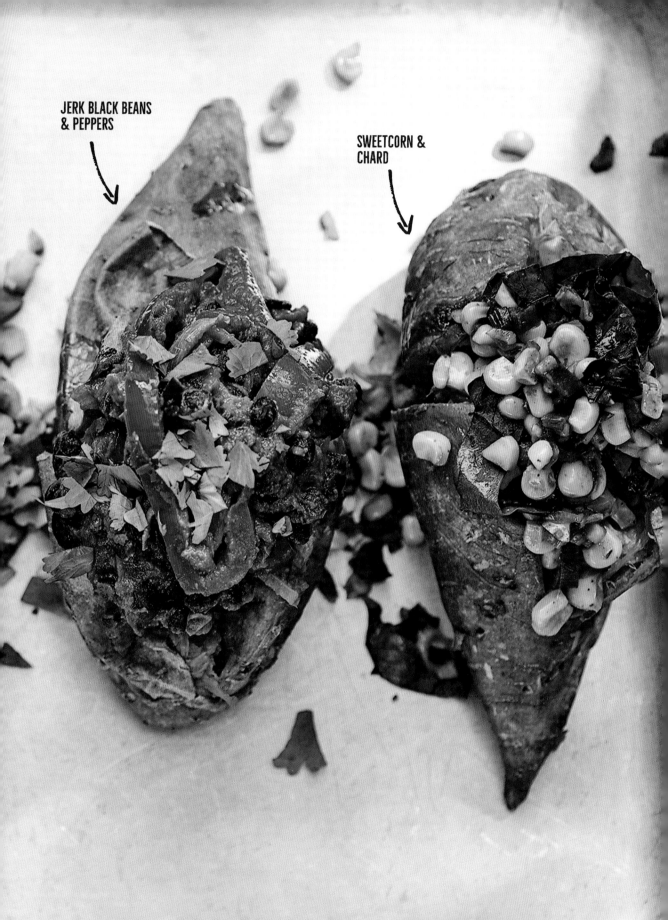

JERK BLACK BEANS
& PEPPERS

SWEETCORN &
CHARD

BEYOND HUMMUS

Traditional hummus is made using chickpeas and is one of my absolute favourites. Here we give you a basic recipe and a few new ideas for equally delicious dips that use a variety of legumes. Serve these on a flatbread (see page 133) with chopped tomatoes and salad greens, or as dips with crunchy veg sticks and wholemeal tortilla chips.

BASIC HUMMUS

Serves 2 as a snack
Prep & cook: 5 minutes

PLANT SCORE: 3
FIBRE PER SERVING: 6.3g
PROTEIN PER SERVING: 10g
GLUTEN-FREE: YES

1 x 400g (14oz) can chickpeas, drained and rinsed

1 tbsp tahini

1 small garlic clove, roughly chopped

1 lemon

Sea salt

1. Put the chickpeas, tahini and garlic into a food processor or blender. Add a good squeeze of lemon juice and blitz until smooth, adding a dash or two of water to thin it to your preferred consistency.

2. Taste and tweak the seasoning with a little salt and more lemon juice to your liking.

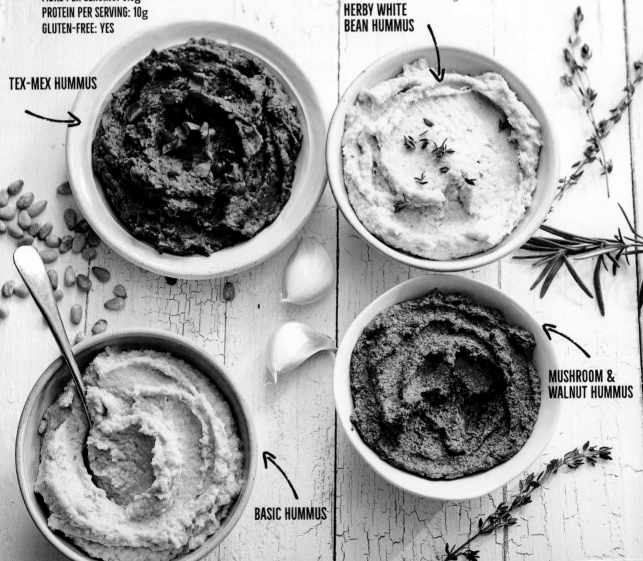

TEX-MEX HUMMUS

HERBY WHITE BEAN HUMMUS

MUSHROOM & WALNUT HUMMUS

BASIC HUMMUS

TEX-MEX HUMMUS

If you're worried about the chilli heat in this recipe, offer the cooling tofu sour cream (see page 86) alongside. This hummus will keep in the fridge for 3–4 days.

Serves 2 as a snack
Prep & cook: 10 minutes

PLANT SCORE: 4
FIBRE PER SERVING: 11g
PROTEIN PER SERVING: 10g
GLUTEN-FREE: YES

1 x 400g (14oz) can black beans, drained and rinsed

2 spring onions, roughly sliced

1 garlic clove, finely chopped

2 tbsp chopped pickled jalapeños, plus 1 tbsp of the pickling liquid

1 tsp ground cumin

Sea salt and lime juice, to taste

Chopped fresh coriander and chilli, to garnish (optional)

1. Put the beans, onions, garlic, jalapeños and cumin in a food processor or blender and blitz until smooth. Taste and add lime juice and sea salt to your liking. Garnish with coriander and a little extra chilli if you want to impress.

2. Serve in a wholewheat wrap or tortilla with some salad leaves, sliced avocado and tomatoes for a quick lunch.

HERBY WHITE BEAN HUMMUS

Cannellini beans, with their relatively thin skin, make for a very smooth hummus. Slather it onto hot toast, topping it with steamed or wilted greens. Store any leftovers in the fridge and use within 3–4 days.

Serves 2 as a snack
Prep & cook: 5 minutes

PLANT SCORE: 3
FIBRE PER SERVING: 10g
PROTEIN PER SERVING: 11g
GLUTEN-FREE: YES

1 x 400g (14oz) can cannellini beans, drained and rinsed (butter beans and haricot beans also work well)

½ tsp fresh thyme leaves

30g (¼ cup) pine nuts

1 garlic clove, finely chopped

1 lemon

Sea salt

1. Place the beans, thyme, pine nuts and half the garlic in a food processor or blender. Add a tablespoon water and a squeeze of lemon juice. Blend to a smooth paste.

2. Taste and tweak with a little sea salt and more garlic and lemon juice to your liking.

MUSHROOM & WALNUT HUMMUS

A little cooking is needed to soften the onions and mushrooms, but after that, this hummus couldn't be easier. The deep mushroom flavour goes beautifully with wholegrain crackers or oatcakes.

Serves 2 as a snack
Prep & cook: 25 minutes

PLANT SCORE: 5
FIBRE PER SERVING: 11g
PROTEIN PER SERVING: 20g
GLUTEN-FREE: YES, IF USING TAMARI RATHER THAN SOY SAUCE

100g (1½ cups) chestnut mushrooms

1 red onion, roughly chopped

1 tbsp extra virgin olive oil (optional)

1 garlic clove

1 tsp finely chopped fresh rosemary leaves

1 x 400g (14oz) can Puy lentils, drained and rinsed

50g (½ cup) walnuts

1 tbsp red wine vinegar, plus more to taste

1 tbsp tamari or soy sauce

Freshly ground black pepper

1. Put the mushrooms and onion into a food processor or blender. Blitz until they appear finely chopped.

2. Warm the oil (if using) or 1 tablespoon water in a non-stick frying pan. Add the mushroom mixture and fry gently for 10–12 minutes, until softened. Add extra dashes of water along the way if it starts to stick. Stir in the garlic and rosemary and cook for a further 2 minutes.

3. Return the mixture to the food processor or blender. Add the lentils, walnuts, vinegar, tamari and a generous twist of black pepper. Blitz until smooth. Add extra seasoning to your taste.

SAVOURY FARINATA

This traditional Italian crêpe is baked in a shallow tray until it sets and starts to colour and blister. If possible, make the batter the night before and leave it to rest in the fridge. The toppings can be made in advance and reheated, or prepared while the farinata is baking.

FARINATA

Serves 2
Prep & cook: 35 minutes + resting time

PLANT SCORE: 1
FIBRE PER SERVING: 5g
PROTEIN PER SERVING: 11g
GLUTEN-FREE: YES

100g (scant 1 cup) chickpea (gram) flour

Pinch of sea salt

300ml (1¼ cups) warm water

Olive oil, for greasing

1. Put the chickpea flour into a mixing bowl with the salt. Whisk in the water until you have a smooth batter. Don't worry if it looks a bit thin and watery, it will thicken when it cooks. Set aside to rest for at least 15 minutes, or ideally overnight in the fridge.

2. Preheat the oven to 200°C/Fan 180°C/400°F/Gas 6. Use a spoon to skim off any foam on top of the batter. Rub a small ovenproof non-stick frying pan or shallow casserole pan with a little olive oil and put it over a high heat. When very hot, pour in the batter and transfer it to the oven. Bake for about 12–15 minutes, or until golden and set.

3. To serve, slide the farinata out of the pan and tear it into quarters. Serve with one of the fillings on the right.

FARINATA WITH COURGETTES, TOMATOES & CAPERS

Serves 2
Prep & cook: 40 minutes

PLANT SCORE: 6
FIBRE PER SERVING: 8.6g
PROTEIN PER SERVING: 15g
GLUTEN-FREE: YES

2 courgettes, cut into 2cm (¾ inch) chunks

200g (1⅓ cups) cherry tomatoes, halved

1 small red onion, sliced

1 tbsp extra virgin olive oil (optional)

2 tbsp capers, roughly chopped

Small handful of fresh basil leaves, torn

Sea salt and freshly ground black pepper

1 cooked farinata, to serve (see page left)

1. Preheat the oven to 200°C/Fan 180°C/400°F/Gas 6. Throw the courgettes, tomatoes and red onions into a roasting tray with the olive oil (if using), and a dash of water. Roast for 25–30 minutes, until everything is soft and starting to colour at the edges.

2. Remove from the oven, throw in the capers and sprinkle with the torn basil. Taste and tweak the seasoning if you wish.

FARINATA WITH MUSHROOMS, SPINACH, GARLIC & CHILLI

Serves 2

Prep & cook: 15 minutes

PLANT SCORE: 9
FIBRE PER SERVING: 6.6g
PROTEIN PER SERVING: 15g
GLUTEN-FREE: YES

½ tbsp extra virgin olive oil (optional)

200g (3 cups) mixed mushrooms, roughly torn or sliced

100g (1 cup) baby spinach

1 garlic clove, finely chopped

Pinch of dried chilli flakes, or a dab of chipotle paste or harissa

1 lemon

1 cooked farinata, to serve (see page 92)

1. Heat the olive oil or 2 tablespoons water in a large non-stick frying pan. When hot, throw in the mushrooms and cook on a high heat for 4–5 minutes, until nicely coloured and cooked through. You might feel the urge to add more oil at the start, but don't: the mushrooms will release liquid as they cook and this will stop them scorching.

2. Reduce the heat and add the spinach, garlic and chilli, stirring until the spinach wilts, which takes just a minute or so. Remove from the heat and add a squeeze of lemon and a twist of pepper. Taste and adjust the seasoning as you wish.

FARINATA WITH MASALA GREEN BEANS, PEAS & SPRING ONIONS

Serves 2

Prep & cook: 25 minutes

PLANT SCORE: 9
FIBRE PER SERVING: 6.6g
PROTEIN PER SERVING: 15g
GLUTEN-FREE: YES

125g (1¼ cups) French beans, trimmed

2 tomatoes, roughly chopped

1 garlic clove, finely chopped

1 green chilli, deseeded and finely chopped

½ tbsp garam masala

½ tsp ground turmeric

200 ml (¾ cup) water

50g (⅓ cup) frozen peas, defrosted

2 spring onions, finely sliced

½ tsp black onion seeds

1 lemon

Small handful of fresh coriander, roughly chopped

TO SERVE

1 cooked farinata (see page 92)

Mango chutney and lime pickle (optional)

1. Place the green beans in a saucepan with the tomatoes, garlic, chilli, garam masala, turmeric and water. Season lightly with salt and cook over a gentle heat for 15–20 minutes, until the beans are tender and the tomatoes have thickened into a rough sauce. Add a dash more water if it looks at all dry.

2. Add the peas, spring onions and onion seeds, and cook for a further 3–4 minutes until the peas are cooked. Finish with a few twists of pepper and a squeeze or two of lemon. Serve garnished with the chopped coriander, and offer the mango chutney and lime pickle separately if you wish.

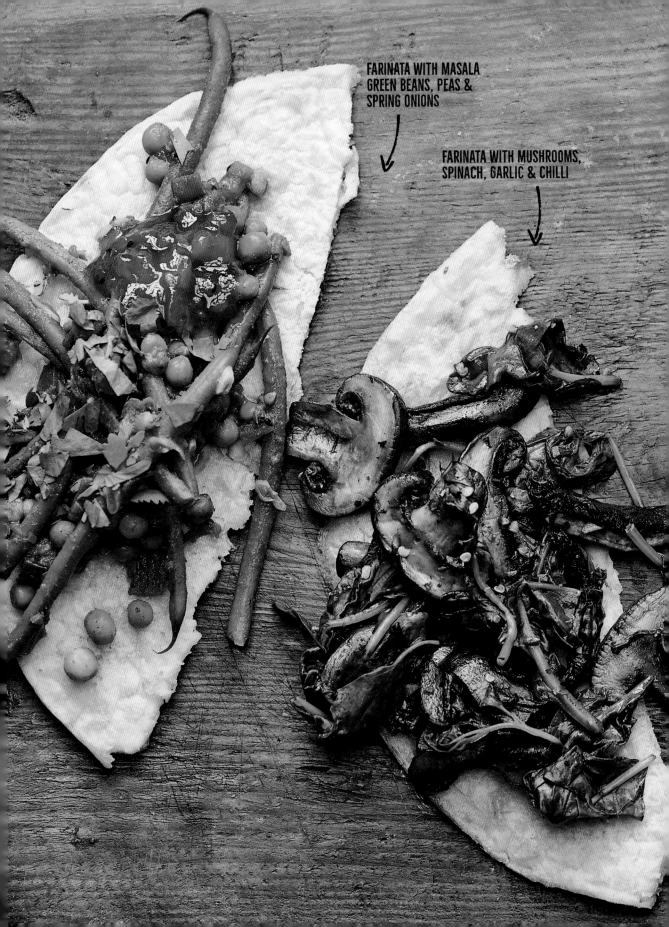

FARINATA WITH MASALA
GREEN BEANS, PEAS &
SPRING ONIONS

FARINATA WITH MUSHROOMS,
SPINACH, GARLIC & CHILLI

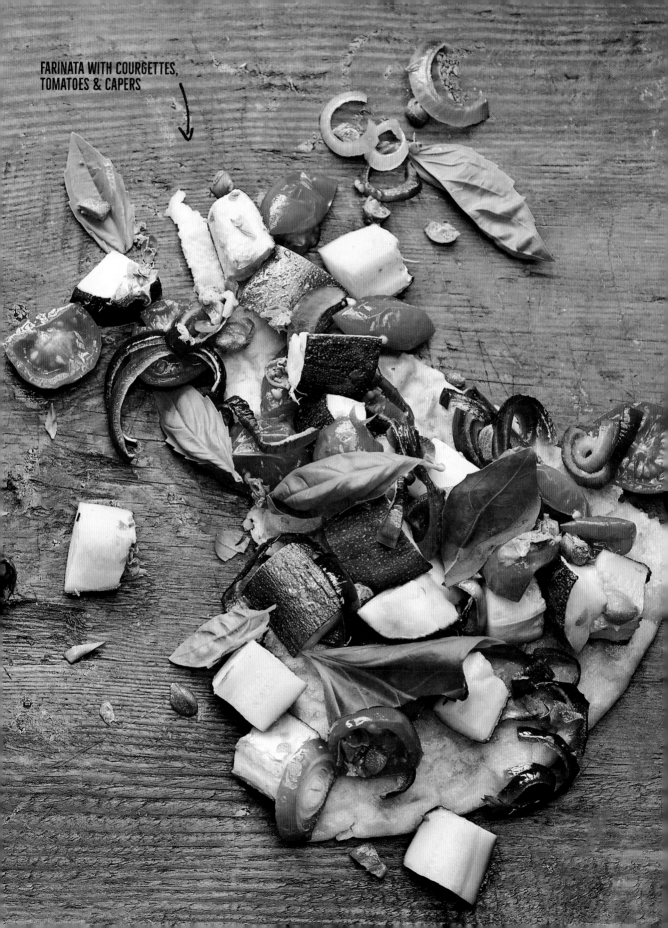

FARINATA WITH COURGETTES,
TOMATOES & CAPERS

FIERY NOODLE SALAD

Thank to a simple but fiery dressing, this beautiful fresh salad packs quite a kick. When preparing the vegetables in this recipe, make sure everything is cut nice and thin, as this will help the dish to carry more of the dressing. A veg peeler makes speedy work of slicing carrots and courgettes into ribbons.

Serves 2
Prep & cook: 20 minutes

PLANT SCORE: 14
FIBRE PER SERVING: 8.8g
PROTEIN PER SERVING: 16g
GLUTEN-FREE: YES, IF USING TAMARI RATHER THAN SOY SAUCE

100g (4oz) buckwheat or brown rice noodles

6 radishes, quartered

50g (½ cup) mangetout, finely sliced

1 carrot, sliced into ribbon-like strips

1 courgette, sliced into ribbon-like strips

2 spring onions, finely sliced

1 small pak choi, broken into leaves and roughly sliced or torn

20g (⅔ cup) sprouted seeds or beans (kale, broccoli, alfalfa or mung)

Small handful of fresh coriander, finely chopped

6 large mint leaves, finely sliced

1 tbsp sesame seeds

FOR THE DRESSING

1 tsp finely grated fresh root ginger

1 small red chilli, deseeded and finely chopped (or retain the seeds if you want extra heat)

1 tbsp peanut butter

2 tbsp tamari or soy sauce

1 tbsp brown rice vinegar

1. Bring a large saucepan of water to the boil and cook the noodles according to the packet instructions.

2. Meanwhile, whisk all the dressing ingredients together in a large bowl, adding a dash of hot water if the mixture seems a bit too thick. Set aside.

3. When the noodles are just done, drain and cool them straight away under cold running water. Drain thoroughly and place them in the bowl of dressing. Add all the vegetables and toss well to combine. Transfer the salad to a large serving plate and garnish with the chopped herbs and sesame seeds.

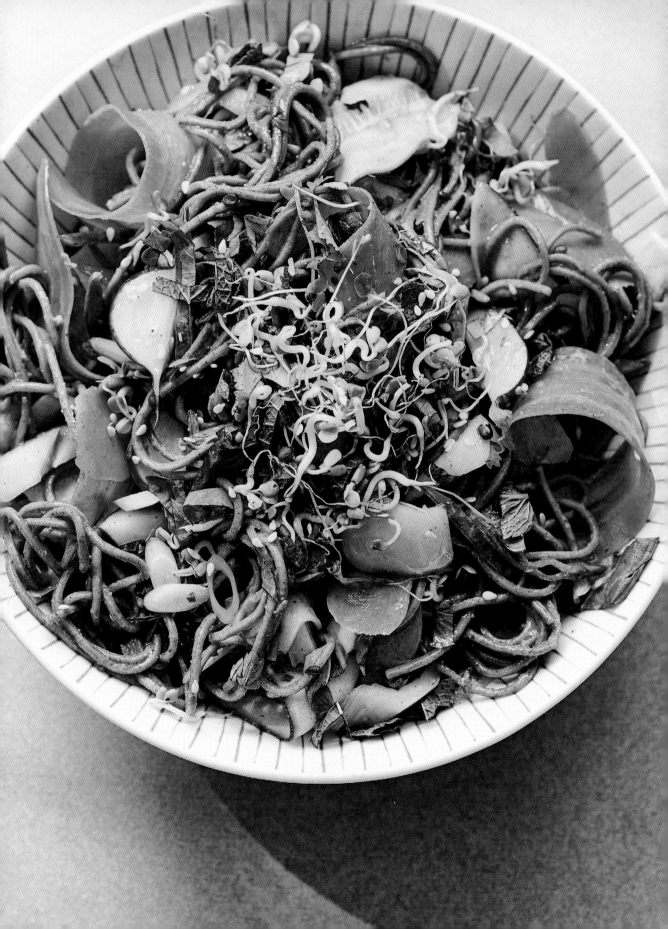

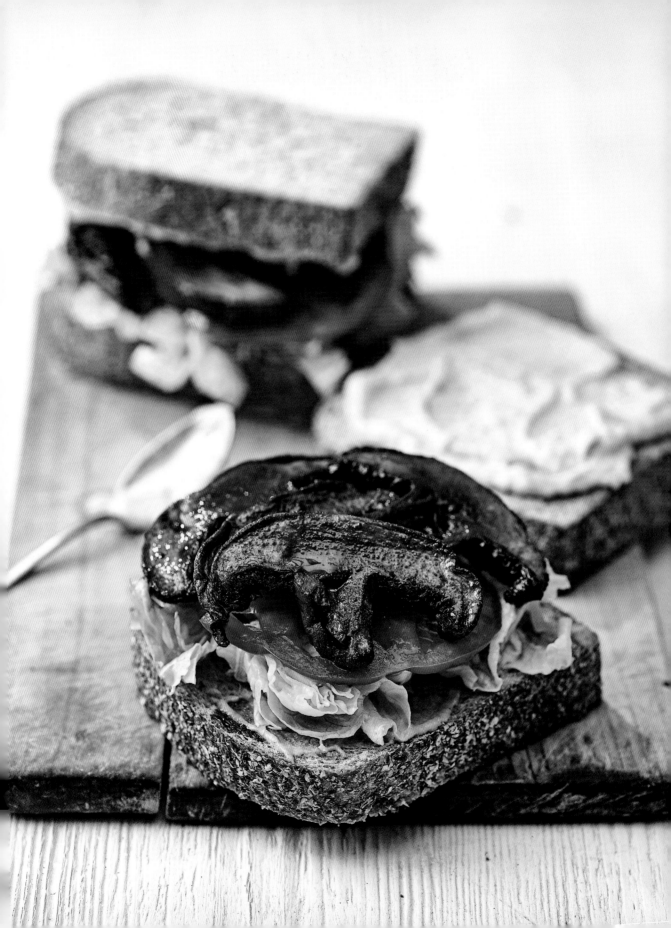

MLT SANDWICH

You'll be surprised by just how meaty and satisfying this mushroom, lettuce and tomato sandwich is. The flavours of the baked mushrooms are definitely big and bold. Adding ripe tomatoes and the cold crunch of fresh lettuce brings you lunchbox perfection.

Makes 2
Prep & cook: 30 minutes

PLANT SCORE: 8
FIBRE PER SERVING: 5.4g
PROTEIN PER SERVING: 7.9g
GLUTEN-FREE: YES, IF USING GLUTEN-FREE BREAD AND TAMARI RATHER THAN SOY SAUCE

2 large Portobello mushrooms, thickly sliced

2 tbsp tamari or soy sauce

½ tbsp smoked paprika

1 tbsp cider vinegar

½ tbsp maple syrup

4 slices wholemeal bread

100g (4oz) hummus (see page 90, or buy ready-made)

Dijon mustard

1 little gem lettuce, roughly shredded

1 large tomato, sliced

1. Preheat the oven to 200°C/Fan 180°C/400°F/Gas 6.

2. Throw the mushrooms into a large bowl and add the tamari, paprika, vinegar and maple syrup. Mix well to coat, then spread them out on a baking tray. Transfer to the oven and cook for 20 minutes, until dark, tender and starting to crisp at the edges.

3. When ready, spread 2 slices of the bread with some hummus and the other 2 with a little mustard. Top the hummus slices with some shredded lettuce and sliced tomato. Cover generously with hot mushrooms, then pop the mustard bread on top.

BEETROOT, SAUERKRAUT & WATERCRESS SANDWICH

Combining a plant score of 8 with a portion of wholegrains and the gut-friendly bacteria of sauerkraut means that your microbiome will love this sandwich just as much as you do.

Makes 2
Prep 10 minutes

PLANT SCORE: 8
FIBRE PER SERVING: 11g
PROTEIN PER SERVING: 17g
GLUTEN-FREE: YES, IF USING GLUTEN-FREE BREAD

150g (5 oz) cooked beetroot

200g (7oz) canned chickpeas, drained and rinsed

½ tsp ground cumin

1 tbsp balsamic vinegar

½ tbsp tahini

4 slices rye bread

4 tbsp sauerkraut, preferably made with red cabbage

¼ cucumber, deseeded and thinly sliced

Small handful of fresh dill, finely chopped

Handful of watercress

Sea salt

1. Put the beetroot, chickpeas, cumin, vinegar and tahini in a food processor or blender and blend until smooth. Taste and lightly adjust the seasoning with salt.

2. Slather 2 slices of rye bread with the beetroot spread. Top with some sauerkraut, cucumber slices, chopped dill and watercress. Cover with the remaining bread and serve. Alternatively, divide the spread and toppings between the 4 slices and serve as open sandwiches.

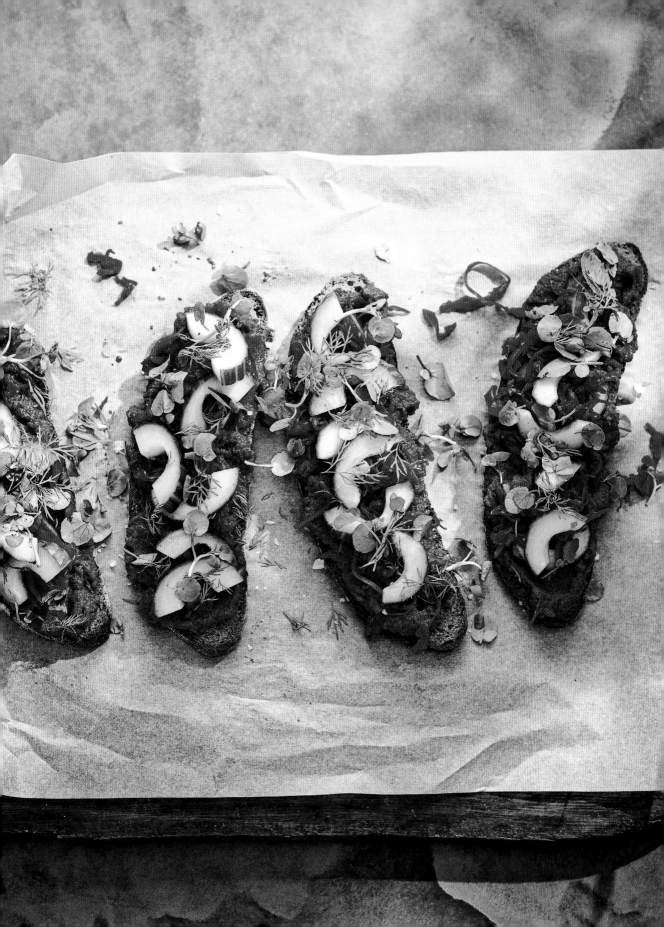

SPICY TOFU ROLLS

These satisfying rolls are ideal for your plant-powered lunchbox. The vegetables need just 10 minutes or so to lightly pickle, making them sharp and sweet with plenty of crunch. Kohlrabi is usually available in the vegetable section throughout the spring and summer. If you can't find kohlrabi, radishes will work just as well in this recipe.

Serves 2
Prep & cook: 25 minutes

PLANT SCORE: 7
FIBRE PER SERVING: 16g
PROTEIN PER SERVING: 44g
GLUTEN-FREE: YES, IF USING GLUTEN-FREE BREAD AND TAMARI RATHER THAN SOY SAUCE

2 tbsp rice vinegar or lime juice

Sea salt

1 spring onion, very finely sliced

1 carrot, coarsely grated or cut into fine matchsticks

¼ head of kohlrabi or 3 radishes, coarsely grated or cut into fine matchsticks

200g (7oz) marinated firm tofu, or marinate slices of plain tofu in tamari or soy sauce overnight

2 small wholegrain baguette rolls

about 4 tbsp crunchy peanut butter

Small handful of fresh coriander, roughly chopped

Ready-made chilli sauce

1. Mix the vinegar and a pinch of salt together in a bowl. Add the onion, carrot and kohlrabi, stir to coat, then set aside to pickle for at least 10 minutes.

2. Cut the tofu into 6 equal slabs. Heat a large non-stick pan, add the tofu and cook for 2–3 minutes on each side, until golden and crisp.

3. Slice the baguette rolls open and spread with the peanut butter. Place 3 slabs of tofu in each roll. Drain the pickled vegetables and divide them between the rolls. Top with some coriander and as much chilli sauce as you like.

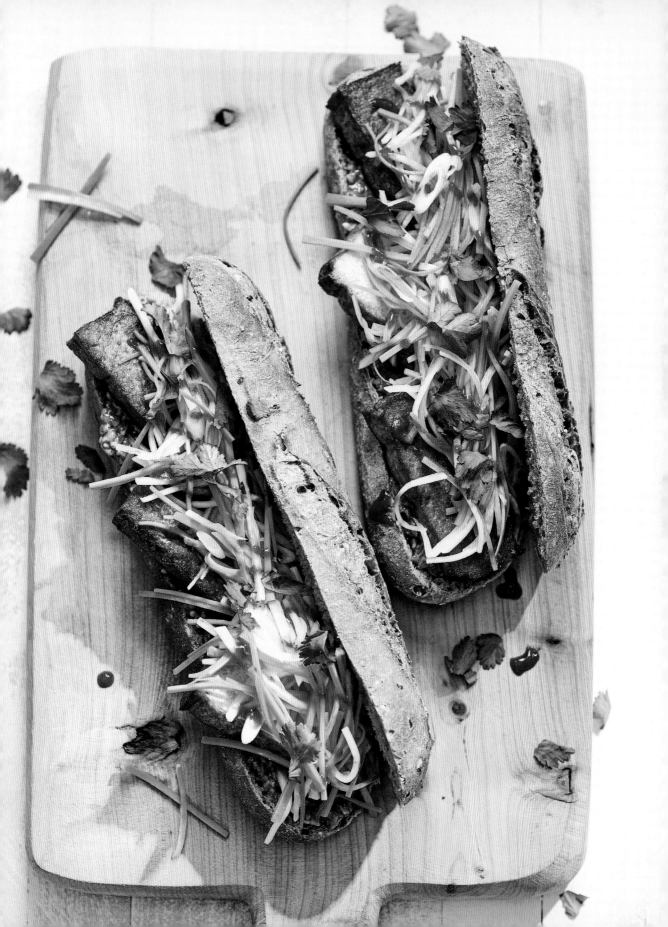

THREE FRESH SLAWS

These slaws make a great addition to any sandwich, wrap or light lunch. Build a quick meal by serving them alongside cooked grains, pulses, rice or noodles, and a few slices of cooked tempeh or tofu.

ALL THE GREENS

Make sure to slice or peel your green veggies as thinly as you can so they carry the dressing well.

Serves 2–4 as a side
Prep: 10 minutes

PLANT SCORE: 8
FIBRE PER SERVING: 7.8g
PROTEIN PER SERVING: 7.4g
GLUTEN-FREE: YES

3 spring onions, finely sliced

1 large courgette, sliced lengthways into thin ribbons

2 celery sticks, finely diced

100g (1 cup) mangetout or French beans, thinly sliced

¼ head of pointed or hispi cabbage, finely sliced

Sea salt and freshly ground black pepper

FOR THE DRESSING

Handful of fresh parsley, finely chopped

6 fresh mint leaves, finely chopped

1 tbsp capers, finely chopped

1 tbsp red wine vinegar

1 tbsp extra virgin olive oil (optional)

1. Combine all the dressing ingredients in a large bowl and mix well.

2. Add all the vegetables and toss to coat.

3. Taste and season to your liking.

FRUIT & ROOT

Either add the oil slowly to the other ingredients, whisking as you go to produce a nice creamy dressing, or put everything in a screwtop jar and shake it up cocktail style. If you prefer an oil-free dressing, use water instead of oil.

Serves 2–4 as a side
Prep: 15 minutes

PLANT SCORE: 6
FIBRE PER SERVING: 12g
PROTEIN PER SERVING: 4.3g
GLUTEN-FREE: YES

1 shallot or ½ red onion, thinly sliced

1 carrot, grated or cut into thin matchsticks

1 parsnip, grated or cut into thin matchsticks

¼ head of Savoy cabbage, finely sliced

1 firm pear, grated or cut into thin matchsticks

30g (3½ tbsp) raisins, roughly chopped

Sea salt and freshly ground black pepper

FOR THE DRESSING

1 tbsp good-quality cider vinegar

1 tsp Dijon mustard

1½ tbsp olive oil or 1 tbsp water

1. To make the dressing, whisk the vinegar and mustard together in a large bowl. Slowly whisk in the oil (if using).

2. Add the vegetables and fruit and toss well. Taste and season to your liking.

ASIAN-STYLE

To keep this slaw nice and crisp, add the dressing just before serving.

Serves 2–4 as a side
Prep: 15 minutes

PLANT SCORE: 9
FIBRE PER SERVING: 6.3g
PROTEIN PER SERVING: 7.8g
GLUTEN-FREE: YES, IF USING TAMARI RATHER THAN SOY SAUCE

3 spring onions, finely sliced

1 large carrot, sliced into long ribbons

¼ head of Chinese cabbage or 1 pak choi, very finely shredded

6 radishes, thinly sliced

Handful of sprouted seeds or beans (kale, broccoli, alfalfa or mung)

1 red chilli, deseeded and finely chopped

Small handful of fresh coriander, finely chopped

25g roasted peanuts, roughly chopped

Sea salt

FOR THE DRESSING

2 tbsp tamari or soy sauce

½ tbsp finely grated fresh root ginger

1 lime

1. To make the dressing, combine the tamari and ginger in a large bowl, then mix in the juice from half the lime.

2. Add all the slaw ingredients and toss well. Season lightly with salt and add more lime juice to taste.

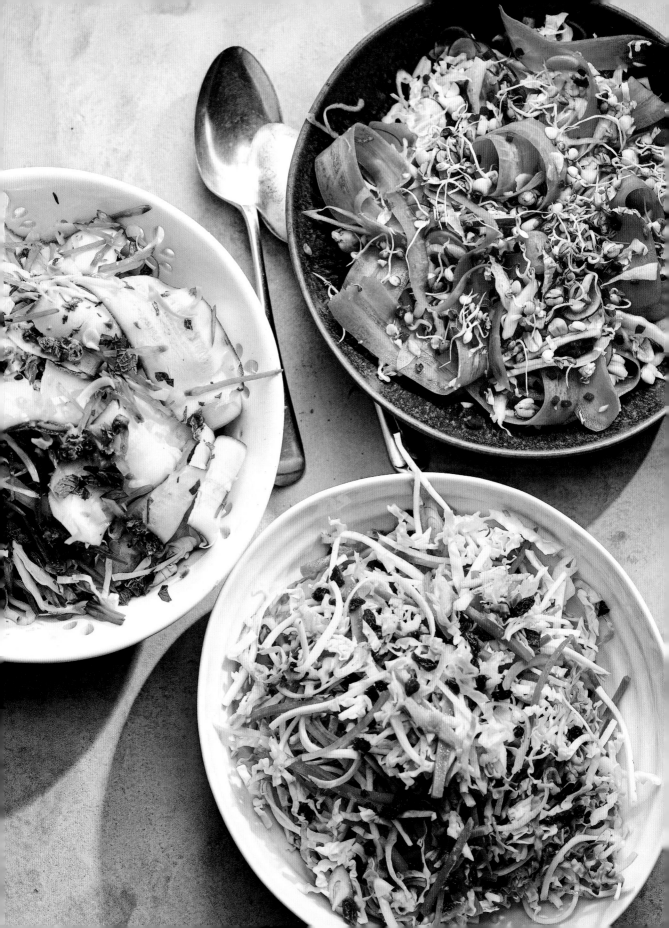

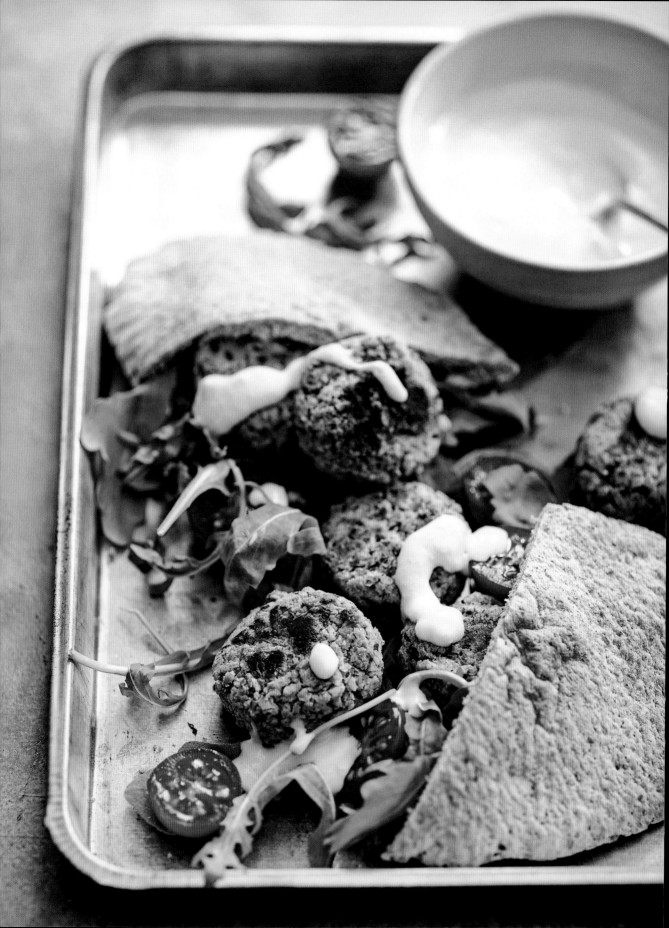

SPEEDY FALAFELS & MORE

These super-quick falafels will be right at home in a warm wholegrain pitta or wrap, with fresh green salad leaves and sliced tomato. Try serving with the tahini dressing on page 132.

Serves 2 – makes about 8
Prep & cook: 15 minutes

PLANT SCORE: 4
FIBRE PER SERVING: 7.6g
PROTEIN PER SERVING: 10g
GLUTEN-FREE: YES

1 x 400g (14oz) can chickpeas, drained and rinsed

1 tsp ground cumin

1 tsp ground coriander

¼ tsp ground cinnamon

Small handful of fresh parsley, stalks removed

1 garlic clove, roughly chopped

1½ tbsp chickpea (gram) flour

1 lemon

1 tbsp extra virgin olive oil (optional)

Sea salt and freshly ground black pepper

1. Preheat the oven to 200°C/Fan 180°C/400°F/Gas 6.

2. Place all the ingredients, apart from the lemon, oil and seasoning, in a food processor or blender. Blitz to a rough paste, then taste and adjust the seasoning to your liking with black pepper, sea salt and lemon juice.

3. Wet your hands and divide the mixture into 8 equal pieces. Roll each one into a ball, then flatten slightly with the palm of your hand.

4. Heat the olive oil (if using) in a non-stick frying pan and cook the falafels for 2 minutes a side, until lightly golden all over. Place them on a baking tray and transfer to the oven to finish cooking for 5 minutes. (If not using the oil, omit the frying and just put them straight on a tray in the oven for 10 minutes.)

VARIATIONS

SPICY FALAFELS

Replace the chickpeas with a can of kidney beans. Add a deseeded red chilli and ½ teaspoon smoked paprika to the mix, and switch the parsley for coriander.

SPEEDY KOFTAS

Replace the chickpeas with a can of Puy lentils. Add 1 tablespoon harissa paste and be prepared to add a bit more chickpea flour if this makes the final mix too wet. Add 5-6 fresh mint leaves along with the parsley.

CHUNKY MINESTRONE

Chunky and satisfying, this minestrone can be adjusted according to the season. In the summertime, try courgettes, tomatoes and chard. For an autumn minestrone, squash and kale will do the trick.

Serves 2
Prep & cook: 45 minutes

PLANT SCORE: 11
FIBRE PER SERVING: 13g
PROTEIN PER SERVING: 13g
GLUTEN-FREE: YES, IF USING GLUTEN-FREE SPAGHETTI

½ tbsp extra virgin olive oil (optional)

1 celery stick, finely diced

1 tomato, roughly chopped

100g (4oz) potatoes, cut into 1cm (½ inch) dice

2 spring onions, finely sliced

1 garlic clove, finely chopped

½ tsp dried thyme

Zest and juice of 1 lemon

200g (7oz) canned cannellini beans, drained and rinsed

500ml (2 cups) vegetable stock

35g (½ cup) wholemeal spaghetti, snapped into 1cm (½ inch) pieces

50g (⅓ cup) podded broad beans

75g (1 cup) spring greens, very finely shredded

100g (4oz) asparagus, thinly sliced

50g (⅓ cup) podded peas, fresh or frozen

Sea salt and freshly ground black pepper

1. Warm the olive oil (if using) or a few tablespoons water in a large saucepan. Add the celery and cook gently over a low heat for 10 minutes, until starting to soften. Add a dash of water every so often if it looks like burning.

2. Add the tomato, potatoes, spring onions, garlic, thyme and lemon zest. Cook for 5 minutes, then add the cannellini beans and stock. Bring to a simmer and cook gently for 10 minutes.

3. Add the spaghetti pieces to the pan, cook for 5 minutes, then add the broad beans and spring greens. Cook for 5 more minutes until the pasta is just tender.

4. Take the pan off the heat, stir in the asparagus and peas, and set aside for a few minutes so the last of the veg cook through.

5. Taste and tweak the seasoning with salt, pepper and a dash or two of lemon juice to taste.

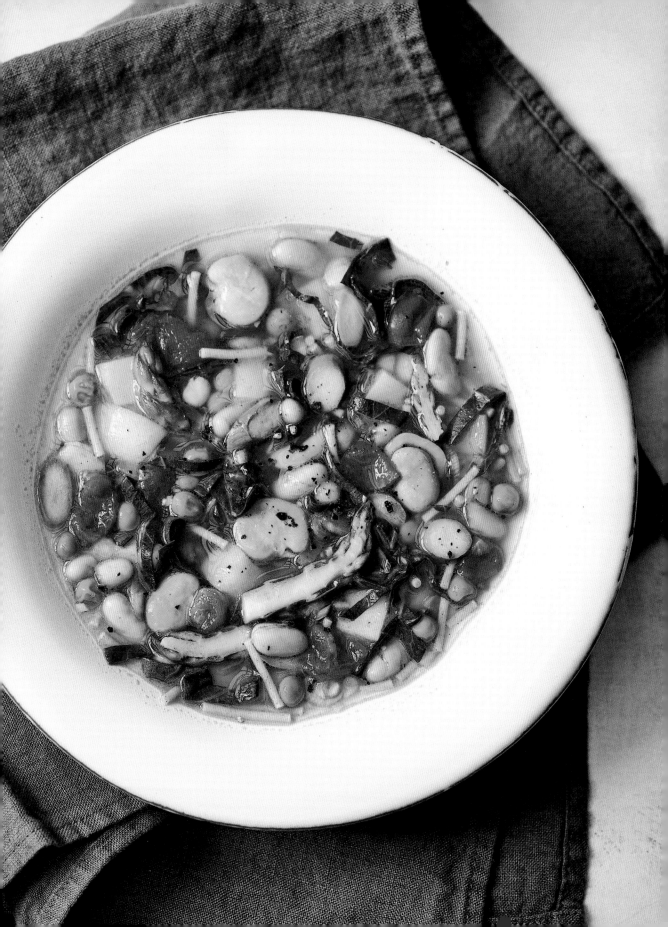

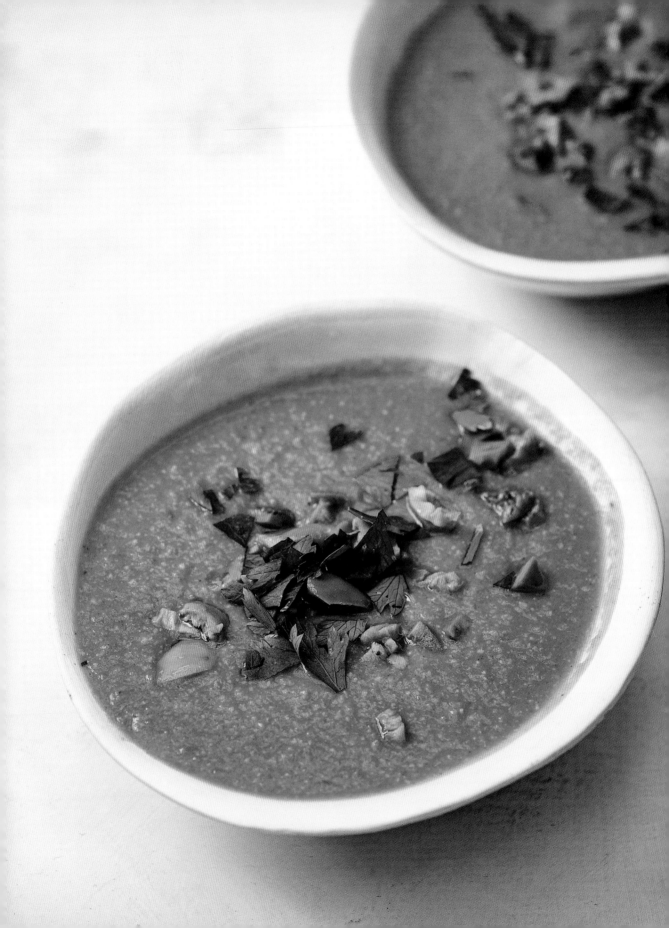

SPANISH RED PEPPER SOUP

This recipe is based on the key ingredients for a Spanish pepper sauce called romesco, which is traditionally thickened with almonds and sometimes a little stale bread. The chickpeas add bulk and protein to make this a more complete meal. You can roast and skin your own peppers, or buy a jar pre-cooked.

Serves 2
Prep & cook: 45 minutes

PLANT SCORE: 9
FIBRE PER SERVING: 11g
PROTEIN PER SERVING: 14g
GLUTEN-FREE: YES

½ tbsp extra virgin olive oil (optional)

1 red onion, sliced

1 celery stick, roughly diced

200g (7oz) canned chickpeas, drained and rinsed

50g (½ cup) flaked and toasted almonds

2 garlic cloves, finely chopped

1 tsp smoked paprika

½ tsp ground cumin

Pinch of dried chilli flakes

1 tbsp red wine vinegar or sherry vinegar, plus extra to taste

200g (7oz) roasted and skinned red peppers

200g (7oz) chopped tomatoes, canned or fresh

400ml (1¾ cups) vegetable stock

Sea salt and freshly ground black pepper

TO SERVE

30g (¼ cup) green olives, roughly chopped

Small handful of fresh parsley, finely chopped

1. Warm the oil (if using) or a few tablespoons water in a large saucepan. Add the onion and celery and cook gently over a low heat for 10 minutes, until starting to soften. Add a dash of water every so often if they look like burning.

2. Add the chickpeas, almonds, garlic, paprika, cumin, chilli and vinegar. Cook for 2 more minutes before adding the peppers, tomatoes and stock. Bring to a simmer and cook for 20 minutes, until everything is tender.

3. Transfer to a blender, in batches if necessary, and whizz until completely smooth. If you like, add some boiling water to adjust the thickness. Taste and tweak the seasoning lightly with salt, pepper and more vinegar.

4. Serve in deep bowls topped with some chopped olives and parsley.

SPICY PARSNIP & LENTIL WINTER SOUP

A perfect winter warmer with ten unique plants in the bowl. Parsnips carry spices beautifully, and their sweetness provides a nice contrast to the earthy lentils. As an alternative to parsnips, you could use carrots, squash, celeriac or sweet potatoes.

Serves 2
Prep & cook: 50 minutes

PLANT SCORE: 10
FIBRE PER SERVING: 15g
PROTEIN PER SERVING: 16g
GLUTEN-FREE: YES

½ tbsp extra virgin olive oil (optional)

1 leek, sliced

1 celery stick, roughly diced

1 tomato, roughly chopped

250g (9oz) parsnips, roughly diced

½ tbsp finely grated fresh root ginger

2 garlic cloves, finely chopped

80g (¾ cup) red lentils, rinsed

1½ tbsp medium-hot curry powder or paste

750ml (3 cups) vegetable stock

1 lemon

Sea salt and freshly ground black pepper

TO SERVE

30g (¼ cup) walnuts, roughly chopped

1 apple, cored and finely diced

Small handful of fresh coriander, finely chopped

1. Warm the oil (if using) or a few tablespoons water in a large saucepan. Add the leek and celery and cook over a low heat for 10 minutes, until starting to soften. Add a dash of water every so often if they look like burning.

2. Add the tomato, parsnips, ginger and garlic. Cook for a further 5 minutes before adding the lentils, curry powder and stock. Bring to a simmer and cook gently for 30 minutes, stirring occasionally, until everything is tender. Stir in a small squeeze of lemon juice.

3. Transfer to a blender, in batches if necessary, and whizz until completely smooth. If you like, add some boiling water to adjust the thickness. Taste and tweak the seasoning with salt, pepper and more lemon juice.

4. Serve in deep bowls topped with the walnuts, apple and coriander.

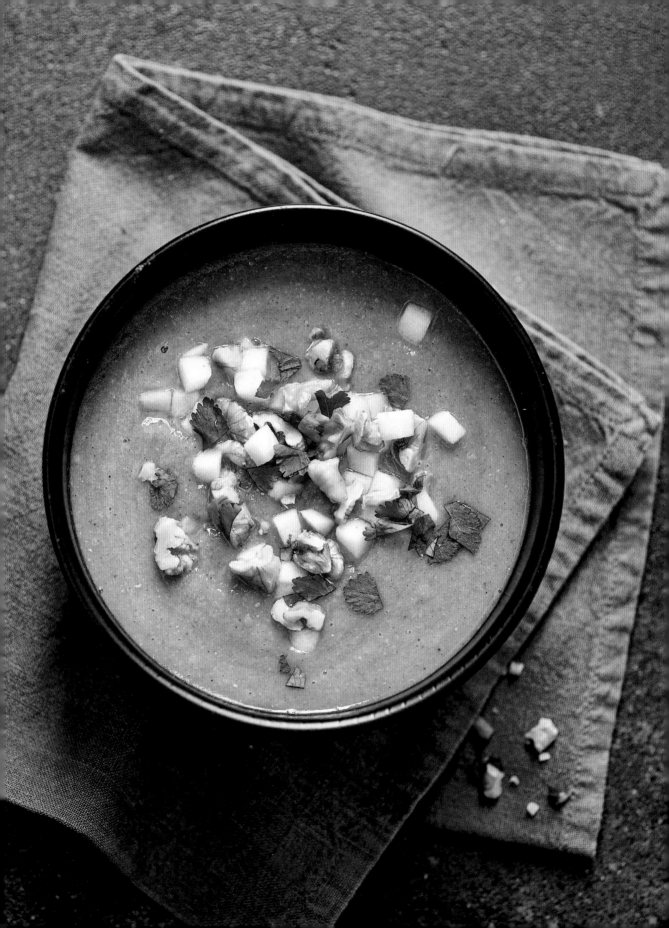

SQUASH & RAW KALE QUINOA SALAD

To make the deliciously creamy dressing you'll need to soak the cashews overnight. Massaging the kale leaves with lemon juice allows them to wilt and tenderise beautifully.

Serves 2
Prep & cook: 40 minutes + overnight soaking

PLANT SCORE: 7
FIBRE PER SERVING: 13g
PROTEIN PER SERVING: 18g
GLUTEN-FREE: YES

1 small autumn squash, deseeded and cut into wedges

1 red onion, sliced

½ tbsp extra virgin olive oil (optional – see tips for roasting without oil, page 60)

100g (⅔ cup) red quinoa

350ml boiling water

1 head of black kale

½ lemon

FOR THE DRESSING

50g ⅓ cup) cashew nuts

Small handful of fresh parsley, roughly chopped

½ garlic clove, finely chopped

1 tsp Dijon mustard

½ lemon

3 tbsp cold water

Sea salt and freshly ground black pepper

1. To make the dressing, put the cashew nuts in a bowl, cover with cold water and leave them to soak in the fridge overnight. The next day, drain them well and place in a food processor or blender with the parsley, garlic, mustard, 1 tablespoon lemon juice and water. Blitz until smooth, scraping down the sides every so often. If the dressing tastes a bit gritty, add a dash more water and blitz again. Season with salt and more lemon juice to your taste.

2. Preheat the oven to 200ºC/ Fan 180ºC/400ºF/Gas 6.

3. Put the squash and onion into a large roasting tray with the olive oil (if using) and about 2 tablespoons cold water. Season lightly with salt and pepper and mix well. Place in the oven and roast for 20–30 minutes, or until the squash is tender and starting to colour at the edges. Set aside until warm or cold, as you prefer.

4. Meanwhile, rinse the quinoa in a sieve under cold running water. Pour the boiling water into a saucepan, add the quinoa and cook gently for 12–15 minutes, until tender. Set aside until warm or cold, as you prefer.

5. While the quinoa cooks, remove and discard the kale stalks. Tear the leaves into bite-sized pieces. Throw them into a large bowl with a good squeeze of lemon juice, then use your hands to massage the leaves for a few minutes.

6. To serve, tumble the squash, onions, quinoa and kale together in a large serving dish. Spoon the dressing over the top.

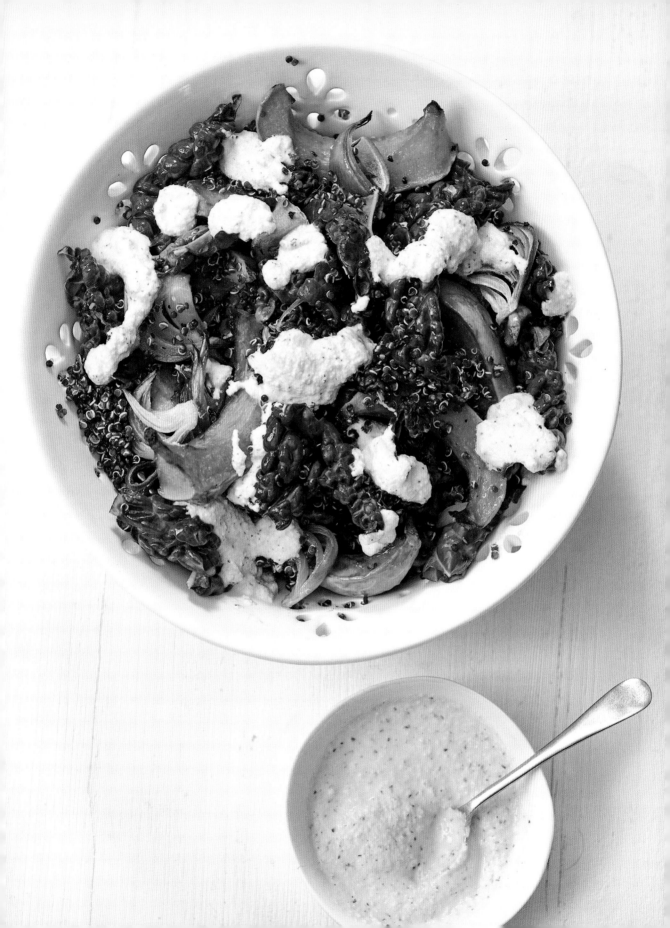

WILD RICE SUPER SALAD

This is a big salad with a lot of components, but it's worth the effort. Alongside the nuts and seeds, the wild rice brings plenty of protein to this dish. You can cook it ahead of time as long as you cool it quickly after cooking and keep it in the fridge.

Serves 2 generously
Prep & cook: 45 minutes

PLANT SCORE: 11
FIBRE PER SERVING: 15g
PROTEIN PER SERVING: 22g
GLUTEN-FREE: YES

150g (scant 1 cup) wild rice, rinsed

¼ head of red cabbage, very finely shredded

½ small red onion, finely sliced

2 beetroot, peeled and cut into fine matchsticks

1 small fennel bulb, trimmed and very finely sliced

2 tbsp red wine vinegar

½ tbsp Dijon mustard

1 apple, cored and diced

1 large handful of radicchio or other bitter leaves, roughly torn

40g (⅓ cup) toasted and chopped hazelnuts or walnuts

Ground allspice, to taste

Small handful of fresh dill, roughly chopped

1 tbsp extra virgin olive oil

30g (⅓ cup) mixed seeds (poppy, pumpkin and sesame are ideal)

Sea salt and freshly ground black pepper

1. Bring a large pan of water to the boil. Add the rice and bring to a simmer. Cook for 35–40 minutes, until tender, topping up with a little more water if and when needed. (Note that wild rice, unlike white rice, has a chewy bite to it when cooked.) When ready, cool in a sieve under cold running water, then set aside to drain.

2. While the rice cooks, combine the cabbage, onion, beetroot and fennel in a large bowl and stir in the vinegar, mustard and a pinch of salt. Set aside to soften.

3. Add the cooled rice to the cabbage mixture along with the apple, radicchio, hazelnuts, allspice and dill. Add the olive oil and a twist of pepper before mixing well.

4. Divide the salad between 2 bowls and finish with a scattering of mixed seeds.

FOR A WARM SALAD:

Oven roast the beetroots in wedges for about 1 hour, Add the fennel, cabbage and shallots for the last 20 minutes, and stir them through the just-cooked rice before adding everything else for the final mix.

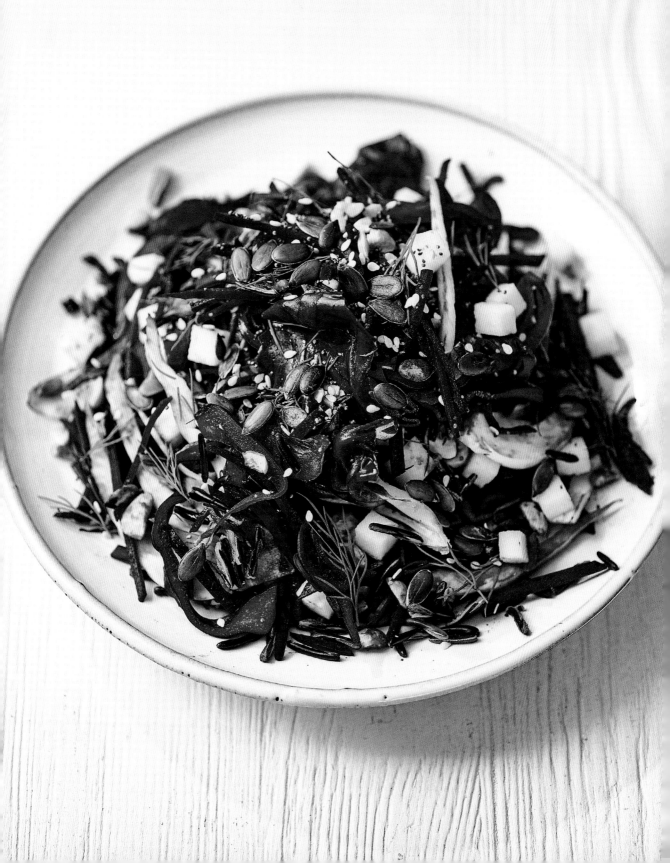

AVOCADO ON TOAST WITH FOUR TWISTS

Avo on toast is a modern classic. Here are four ways to reinvent this plant-based favourite. Each version will work nicely with the Brown soda bread on page 71, sliced thinly and toasted, or with any good wholemeal bread.

AVOCADO TOAST WITH RADISH & SPROUTED SEEDS

Perfect if the radishes have got a nice hot kick to them. The sprouted beans or seeds will add some protein as well as texture.

Serves 2 • Prep: 15 minutes

PLANT SCORE: 6
FIBRE PER SERVING: 8.5g
PROTEIN PER SERVING: 8.1g
GLUTEN-FREE: YES, IF USING GLUTEN-FREE BREAD

4 radishes, very thinly sliced

1 tbsp rice or red wine vinegar

2 large slices of wholemeal bread

Flesh from 2 avocados

Handful of pea shoots, watercress or lamb's lettuce

1 spring onion, very finely sliced

Small handful of sprouted seeds or beans (kale, broccoli, alfalfa or mung are ideal)

Sea salt and freshly ground black pepper

1. Place the radishes in a bowl with the vinegar and a pinch of sea salt. Mix well, then set aside for 10 minutes to lightly pickle.

2. Toast the bread and slice the avocados. Divide the pea shoots between the toast and top them with sliced avocado. Add salt and pepper to taste.

3. Remove the radishes from the vinegar and scatter them over the avocado, followed by some spring onions and sprouted seeds.

AVOCADO PESTO TOAST WITH TOMATOES

My favourite version of avocado on toast, this is ideal for a summer's day, when the basil and tomatoes should be at their best.

Serves 2 • Prep & cook: 5 minutes

PLANT SCORE: 6
FIBRE PER SERVING: 8.5g
PROTEIN PER SERVING: 12g
GLUTEN-FREE: YES, IF USING GLUTEN-FREE BREAD

Flesh from 2 avocados

Small handful of fresh basil

1 tbsp pine nuts

1 tbsp nutritional yeast

1 small garlic clove, finely chopped

1 lemon

2 large slices of bread

200g (7oz) tomatoes, sliced

Sea salt and freshly ground black pepper

1. Put the avocado, basil, pine nuts, nutritional yeast and garlic in a food processor or blender with a squeeze of lemon. Blitz together, then tweak the seasoning to your liking.

2. Toast the bread and slather each slice with the avocado pesto. Top with slices of tomato and season with salt and pepper to taste.

AVOCADO TOAST WITH MISO 'SHROOMS & SESAME SEEDS

This is another great way to unleash the savoury taste of mushrooms. Miso ramps up their natural savouriness, making these 'shrooms dark, sticky and incredibly tasty.

Serves 2 • Prep & cook: 15 minutes

PLANT SCORE: 6
FIBRE PER SERVING: 10g
PROTEIN PER SERVING: 10g
GLUTEN-FREE: YES, IF USING GLUTEN-FREE BREAD

½ tbsp extra virgin olive oil (optional)

150g (2 cups) mushrooms, ideally shiitake, sliced

1 tbsp sweet white miso paste

1 garlic clove, finely chopped

2 tbsp water

1 lemon

2 large slices of wholemeal bread

Flesh from 2 avocados

1 tbsp sesame seeds

1. Heat the olive oil (if using) or a few tablespoons water in a large frying pan. Throw in the mushrooms and fry for 5 minutes, until they are cooked and starting to colour.

2. Add the miso, garlic and water and cook for a further 3 minutes, until the water has evaporated and the mushrooms are dark and sticky. Finish with a good squeeze of lemon juice and remove from the heat.

3. Toast the bread. Slice the avocados and divide them between the toast. Top with the warm mushrooms and garnish with sesame seeds.

GUACAMOLE TOAST WITH POPPED BEANS

Roasting the beans gives them some texture and extra flavour and acts as a contrast to the clean sharp flavour in the guacamole.

Serves 2 • Prep & cook: 15 minutes

PLANT SCORE: 6
FIBRE PER SERVING: 14g
PROTEIN PER SERVING: 12g
GLUTEN-FREE: YES, IF USING GLUTEN-FREE BREAD

200g canned black beans, drained and rinsed

Flesh from 2 avocados

Juice of ½ lime

1 small red chilli, deseeded and finely chopped

½ garlic clove, finely chopped

½ tsp ground cumin

2 large slices of bread

Small handful of fresh coriander, roughly chopped

½ tsp smoked paprika

Sea salt

1. Preheat the oven to 200°C/Fan 180°C/400°F/Gas 8.

2. Lay the beans on some kitchen paper or a clean tea towel and gently pat them dry. Spread them out on a baking tray and season with a pinch of salt. Transfer to the oven and roast for 10–12 minutes, until the skins have burst and are starting to crisp a little.

3. Meanwhile, put the avocado flesh into a bowl with the lime juice, chilli, garlic and cumin. Mash with a fork until it becomes a coarse but spreadable mixture. You just made guacamole!

4. Toast the bread and slather each slice with the guacamole. Divide the warm popped beans between the slices and top with some chopped coriander and an artistic dusting of paprika.

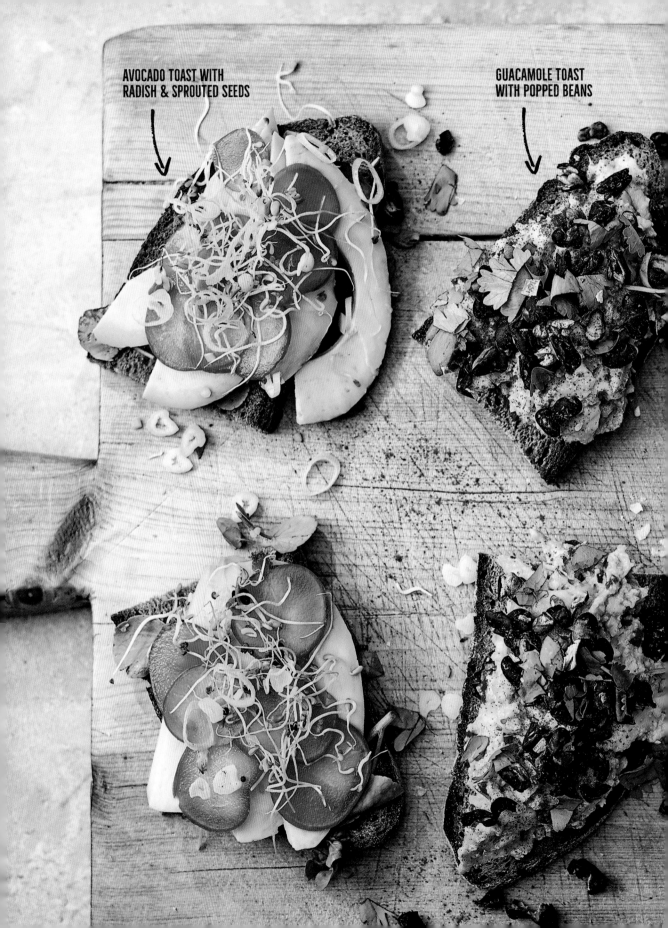

AVOCADO TOAST WITH
RADISH & SPROUTED SEEDS

GUACAMOLE TOAST
WITH POPPED BEANS

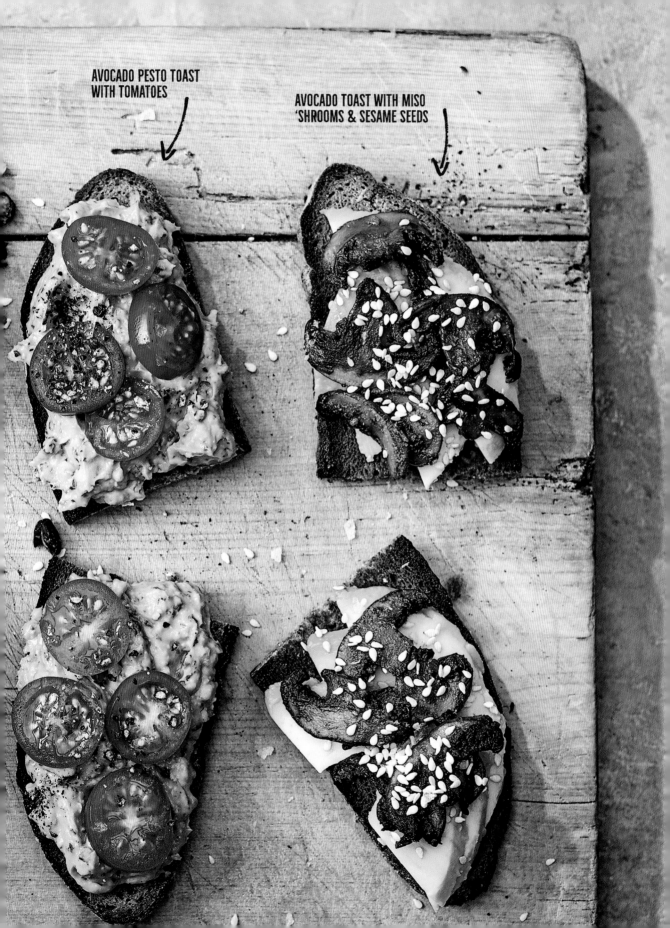

AVOCADO PESTO TOAST
WITH TOMATOES

AVOCADO TOAST WITH MISO
'SHROOMS & SESAME SEEDS

MAIN MEALS

Hearty bolognese with squash & rosemary polenta 124

Rosti pie with braised cabbage & peas 126

Corn & squash spelt risotto with black kale 128

Crispy tofu tacos & chopped salsa salad 130

Lebanese lentil & tahini pittas 132

Plant-powered stew with braised chickpeas & couscous 134

Squash & lemongrass noodle broth 136

Stuffed peppers with artichokes, fennel and farro 138

Summer veg & white bean pasta 140

Tempeh miso stir-fry 142

Winter barley stew with Irish Stout & herby dumplings 144

Sticky tofu, courgettes, greens & kimchi 146

Squash & olive tagine with freekeh 148

Roasting tray ratatouille gratin 150

Sweet potato Massaman curry 152

Cauliflower, butter bean & chard dahl 154

Cajun beans and greens 156

Spanish rice with fennel, tomato and onions 157

Winter pilaf 158

Goulash hotpot 160

Pakora bean burgers with raita & sweet potato chips 162

One-pot chilli bowl 164

Epic nut roast with onion miso gravy 166

Miso aubergines with tofu fried rice 168

Tahini cauliflower with Greek bulgur wheat 170

Autumn roasting tray tempeh 172

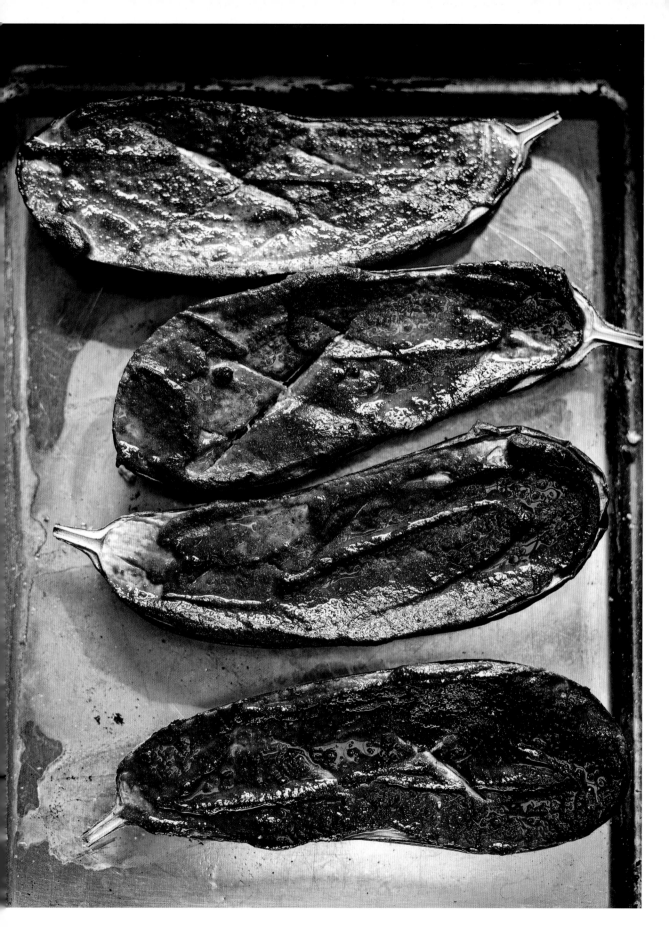

HEARTY BOLOGNESE WITH SQUASH & ROSEMARY POLENTA

This dish is definitely hearty! This Bolognese goes beautifully with the polenta, but of course can always be served with wholewheat spaghetti if you're pushed for time. Grating and braising the squash keeps everything in one pan, but you could oven-roast it in chunks for a deeper taste, stirring it into the dish before serving.

Serves 2
Prep & cook: 50 minutes

PLANT SCORE: 9
FIBRE PER SERVING: 28g
PROTEIN PER SERVING: 37g
GLUTEN-FREE: YES, IF USING TAMARI RATHER THAN SOY SAUCE

1 tbsp extra virgin olive oil (optional)

1 red onion, finely diced

1 celery stick, finely diced

1 carrot, finely diced

100g (1½ cups) chestnut mushrooms, roughly chopped

200g (7oz) tempeh, roughly chopped

2 garlic cloves, finely chopped

1 bay leaves

½ tsp dried oregano

125ml (½ cup) white wine

1 tbsp tamari or soy sauce

1 x 400g (14oz) can chopped tomatoes

Sea salt and freshly ground black pepper

FOR THE POLENTA

300g (11oz) squash, coarsely grated

½ tbsp freshly chopped rosemary leaves

500ml (2 cups) vegetable stock

75g (½ cup) quick-cook polenta

2 tbsp nutritional yeast

1. Warm the olive oil (if using) or a few tablespoons water in a large saucepan and cook the onion, celery and carrot over a medium-low heat for 10 minutes, until starting to soften. Add a dash more water if the veg look like catching at any point.

2. Add the mushrooms and tempeh and cook for another 8 minutes, until they have both taken on a little colour. Stir in the garlic, bay, oregano and wine and cook for 2 minutes before adding the tamari and tomatoes. Add water to the empty tomato can until it's a third full and tip that in too. Bring to a simmer, season lightly with salt and pepper, and cook gently for 20 minutes, until you have a thick rich sauce.

3. Meanwhile, start making the polenta. Put the grated squash in a clean saucepan along with the rosemary and half the stock. Bring to a simmer and cook very gently for 10–15 minutes, until the squash is completely tender and most of the liquid has disappeared.

4. Add the rest of the stock and bring back to a simmer. Pour in the polenta and cook for 2–3 minutes, stirring continuously, until it thickens and starts to pull away from the side of the pan. You don't want it to be too thick, so (as brands vary) you might need to add a dash more water or a little extra cooking time. When it's ready, stir in the nutritional yeast.

5. Serve the polenta in shallow bowls and spoon over the sauce. If you want to offer some greens, a simple side dish of wilted kale, spinach or chard would be ideal.

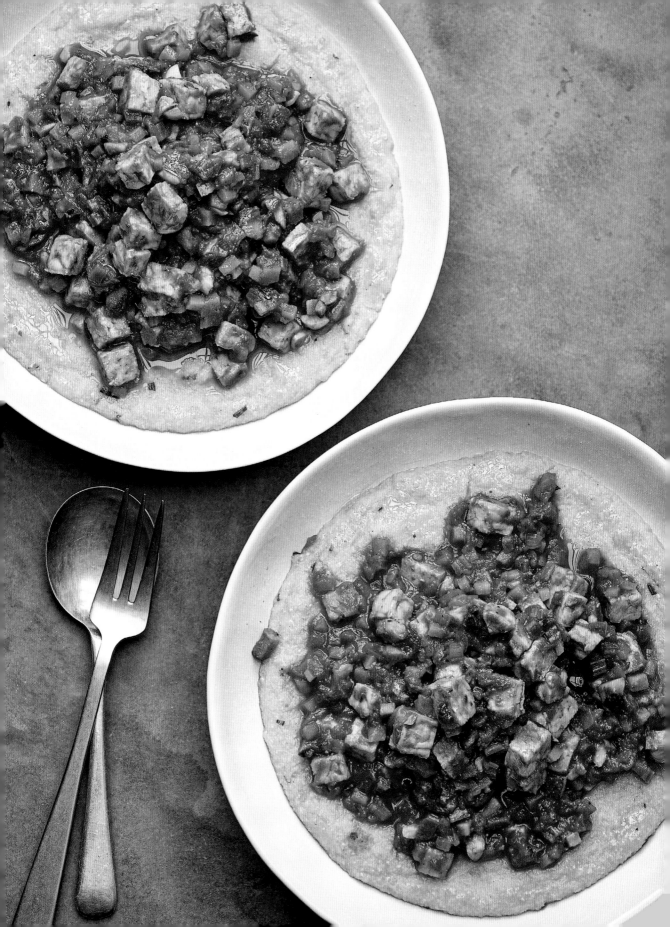

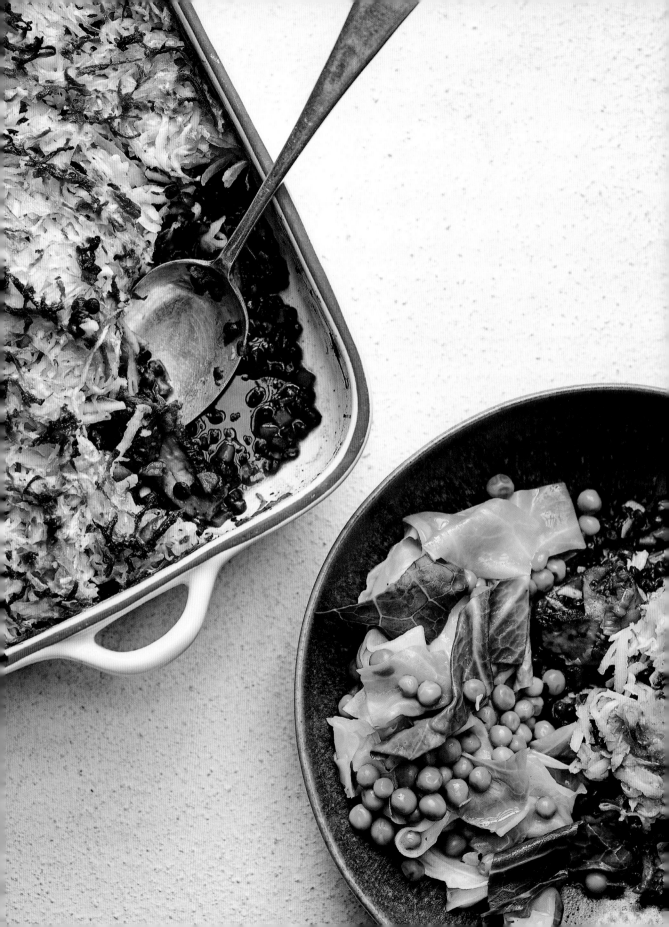

ROSTI PIE WITH BRAISED CABBAGE & PEAS

Combining the comfort of a cottage pie with the crispy edges of a rosti, this recipe is pure pie genius.

Serves 2
Prep & cook: 1 hour

PLANT SCORE: 11
FIBRE PER SERVING: 22g
PROTEIN PER SERVING: 24g
GLUTEN-FREE: YES, IF USING TAMARI RATHER THAN SOY SAUCE

1 tbsp extra virgin olive oil (optional)

1 onion, finely sliced

1 celery stick, finely diced

1 carrot, finely diced

200g (3 cups) Portobello or wild mushrooms, sliced

2 garlic cloves, finely chopped

1 tsp finely chopped rosemary leaves

1 bay leaf

100ml (½ cup) red wine

1 x 400g (14oz) can Puy lentils, drained and rinsed

1 tbsp tamari or soy sauce

400ml (1¾ cups) vegetable stock

FOR THE ROSTI TOPPING

1 potato

½ head of celeriac

1 tbsp Dijon mustard

½ tbsp extra virgin olive oil (optional)

Sea salt and freshly ground black pepper

TO SERVE

½ head of pointed cabbage or a small green cabbage, thickly sliced

100g (¾ cup) frozen peas

1. Preheat the oven to 200ºC/Fan 180ºC/400ºF/Gas 6.

2. First make the topping. Peel and coarsely grate the potato and celeriac into a mixing bowl. Add a pinch of salt, mix well and set aside while you make the filling.

3. Warm the oil (if using) or a few tablespoons water in a non-stick saucepan. Add the onion, celery and carrots and cook over a medium heat for 5 minutes.

4. Add the mushrooms and cook for a further 5 minutes, until they have started to darken and soften.

5. Stir in the garlic, rosemary, bay leaf and wine and allow to bubble away until the wine has reduced by half; this will take only a few minutes.

6. Tip in the lentils, tamari and half the stock. Simmer gently for 10 minutes, until everything is warmed through and tender.

7. Transfer the lentil mixture to an ovenproof dish (about 25 x 25cm) and level the surface with the back of a spoon.

8. To finish the topping, tip the potato mixture into a clean cloth or tea towel, then hold it over the sink and squeeze out as much excess water as you can. Return it to the bowl and mix in the mustard and olive oil (if using).

9. Spoon the topping over the lentils without pressing it down too firmly; the look you're aiming for is scruffy but even. Place in the oven for 20–25 minutes, until the top is golden and the potato cooked through.

10. When the pie is halfway through cooking, place the cabbage in a frying pan with the remaining stock and bring to a simmer over a medium heat. Cook gently for 10 minutes, by which time the cabbage will be tender and most of the stock will have evaporated. Add the peas and cook for 2–3 more minutes. Finish with plenty of freshly ground pepper and serve alongside the pie.

CORN & SQUASH SPELT RISOTTO WITH BLACK KALE

An ideal recipe for the late summer and early autumn, when sweetcorn and squash are at their best. The wholegrain used here is spelt, broken up in a food processor or blender to make the grains more absorbent, but pearled spelt or traditional risotto rice can be used instead.

Serves 2
Prep & cook: 50 minutes

PLANT SCORE: 8
FIBRE PER SERVING: 17g
PROTEIN PER SERVING: 20g
GLUTEN-FREE: YES, IF USING TRADITIONAL RISOTTO RICE INSTEAD OF SPELT

1 large fresh corn cob, or 125g (½ cup) canned corn kernels

150g (1½ cups) wholegrain spelt

1 tbsp extra virgin olive oil (optional)

1 small onion, finely diced

1 celery stick, finely diced

300g (2 cups) squash, cut into 1cm (½ inch) dice

1 garlic clove, finely chopped

½ tsp fresh thyme leaves, plus a few extra to garnish

100ml (½ cup) white wine, or 1½ tbsp cider vinegar

600ml (2½ cups) hot vegetable stock

120g (4½oz) black kale

2 tbsp nutritional yeast

1 lemon

Sea salt and freshly ground black pepper

FOR THE GARNISH

2 tbsp toasted pumpkin seeds

½ tsp dried chilli flakes

Dash of extra virgin olive oil

1. If using fresh sweetcorn, remove and discard any husks. Stand the cob upright and slice down the sides to remove the kernels. Don't waste the spent cob; if added to the pan of stock, it will impart some of its flavour as it warms up.

2. Put the spelt grains in a food processor or blender and pulse a few times to crack them open. Don't overblend, as you want them to be coarse.

3. Warm the olive oil (if using) or a few tablespoons water in a non-stick saucepan. Add the onion and celery and cook gently for 5 minutes, until starting to soften, adding a dash more water every so often if they start to catch.

4. Add the sweetcorn and squash and cook for a further 8 minutes, stirring occasionally and adding extra water if needed.

5. Throw in the garlic, thyme and spelt and cook for 2 more minutes before tipping in the wine. Let it bubble away until it seems to have been absorbed by the grain. If using cider vinegar instead, don't wait for it to reduce – just go straight to adding the stock.

6. Bring the pan to a medium heat and add a ladleful of hot stock. Cook gently, stirring occasionally, until the stock has been absorbed. Repeat this step, adding the stock a ladleful at a time until the spelt is tender; this will take about 30 minutes.

7. Meanwhile, cut out and discard the kale stalks, then roughly chop the leaves. Put them in a saucepan with a dash of water and cook over a gentle heat for 10 minutes, until completely wilted and tender. Add a dash more water if they look like drying out. Set aside until needed.

8. When the spelt is ready, stir in the nutritional yeast. Taste and tweak the seasoning to your liking with salt and pepper and a squeeze of lemon juice . Set aside for 5 minutes while you make the garnish.

9. Roughly chop the pumpkin seeds and mix them with the chilli and extra thyme leaves. Add a very small dash of oil, just enough to bind the ingredients.

10. Serve the risotto in shallow bowls topped with a pile of wilted kale. Sprinkle with the garnish and finish with a few fresh twists of black pepper.

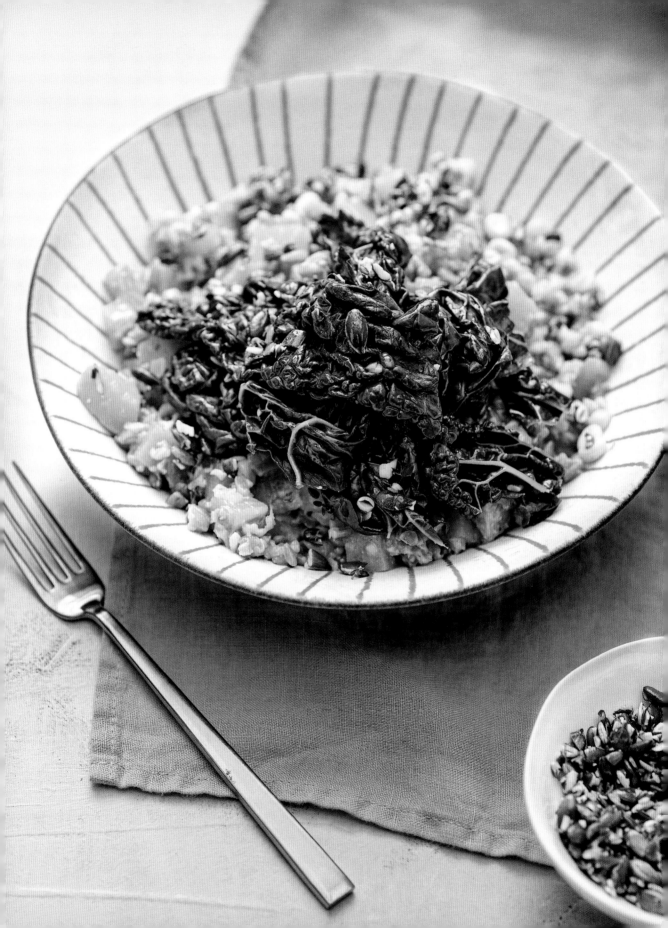

CRISPY TOFU TACOS & CHOPPED SALSA SALAD

Baking the tofu rather than frying it uses far less oil to get the perfect level of crispness. You can whisk or mash the avocado dressing with a fork, but using a blender will guarantee a super-smooth result.

Serves 2
Prep & cook: 30 minutes

PLANT SCORE: 10
FIBRE PER SERVING: 12g
PROTEIN PER SERVING: 27g
GLUTEN-FREE: YES, IF USING GLUTEN-FREE WRAPS OR TORTILLAS

200g (7oz) firm or extra firm tofu, cut into 1cm (½ inch) dice

½ tbsp ground cumin

1 tsp ground coriander

¼ tsp ground cinnamon

2 tbsp cornflour

2 tomatoes, roughly chopped

⅓ cucumber, deseeded and finely diced

½ small red onion, finely diced

1 little gem lettuce, roughly chopped

2 tbsp finely chopped pickled jalapeños, or 1 chopped fresh chilli

Small handful of fresh coriander, finely chopped

½ tbsp extra virgin olive oil (optional)

4 corn or wholemeal tortillas (15cm/ 6 inch diameter), or homemade flatbreads (see page 133)

Sea salt and freshly ground black pepper

Hot chilli sauce, to serve (optional)

FOR THE DRESSING

1 large avocado, stoned and peeled

½ garlic clove, finely chopped

Juice of 1 lime

1. Preheat the oven to 200°C/Fan 180°C/ 400°F/Gas 6. Place the diced tofu in a bowl, sprinkle in the spices, cornflour and a pinch of salt and pepper. Mix with your fingers to coat, taking care not to break up the tofu too much. Transfer to a baking tray and bake for 20 minutes, turning halfway through, until golden and crisp.

2. Meanwhile, put the tomatoes, cucumber, onion and lettuce in a bowl, adding the jalapeños, coriander, olive oil (if using) and a pinch of salt. Mix gently, then set aside.

3. To make the dressing, put the avocado, garlic and 1 tablespoon of the lime juice into a food processor or blender and blitz until smooth. Add some cold water, a little at a time, until the mixture has a pourable yogurt-like consistency. Season lightly with salt and more lime to taste.

4. When the tofu is ready, warm the tortillas in the oven for a couple of minutes. Pile some chopped salad into each one and divide the tofu equally between them. Spoon over some avocado dressing and a zigzag of chilli sauce, if using. Fold in half and eat immediately.

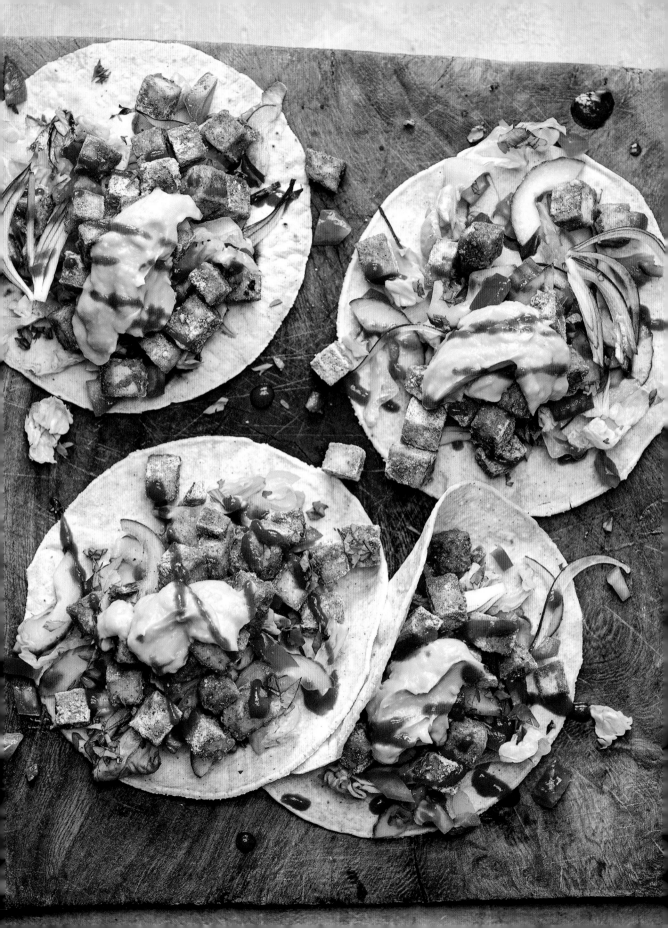

LEBANESE LENTIL & TAHINI PITTAS

This legume-powered dish is wonderfully filling and is a great meal to share. Serve with a portion of wholegrain rice, or with the simple wholemeal flatbreads below.

Serves 2
Prep & cook: 40 minutes

PLANT SCORE: 13
FIBRE PER SERVING: 17g
PROTEIN PER SERVING: 24g
GLUTEN-FREE: YES, IF USING GLUTEN-FREE PITTA BREADS

1 x 400g (14oz) can Puy lentils, drained

1 garlic clove, finely chopped

1 tbsp tomato purée

1 green chilli, finely chopped

30g (3½ tbsp) sultanas, chopped

1 tbsp bahrat spice mix, or make your own (1 tsp each ground cumin, coriander and paprika, and a pinch each of ground cinnamon and clove)

1 lemon

6 fresh mint leaves, chopped

Small handful of fresh coriander, chopped

FOR THE DRESSING

3 tbsp light tahini

1 tbsp lemon juice

2 tbsp boiling water

Sea salt

TO SERVE

2 wholemeal pitta breads or homemade flatbreads (see opposite)

1 tomato, sliced

⅓ cucumber, deseeded and thinly sliced

½ small red onion, thinly sliced

Handful of watercress or mixed salad leaves

1. To make the dressing, mix the tahini with the lemon juice. Whisk in the boiling water to make a thick, yogurt-like consistency, adding more water if needed. Season to taste with salt.

2. Put the lentils in a frying pan with the garlic, tomato purée, chilli, sultanas and spice mix. Stir it all together, then cook on a gentle heat for 10 minutes, until the water has almost evaporated.

3. Increase the heat and fry for a few more minutes, until the lentils start to dry out and catch on the bottom of the pan. Remove from the heat and add a squeeze of lemon juice. Taste and tweak the seasoning with salt and lemon juice to your liking. Stir the mint and coriander in to finish.

4. Warm up the pittas, then slice them open to form pockets. Tuck some tomato, cucumber, onion and watercress into each one, followed by the warm lentils. Finish with a streak of tahini dressing.

WHOLEMEAL FLATBREADS

These couldn't be easier: if you can knead dough and use a rolling pin you can't fail. The heat from the dry pan cooks them quickly, blistering the outsides. For a quick breakfast serve these straight from the pan with a simple fruit compote (page 68) or a generous spreading of nut butter (page 72). They'll also do as an added side if you're having spring tofu hash (page 76) or baked kedgeree (page 82) for breakfast! The breads can be used hot or cold.

Makes 2
Prep & cook: 20 minutes

FIBRE PER SERVING: 3.8g
PROTEIN PER SERVING: 4.5g
GLUTEN-FREE: NO

75g (½ cup) wholemeal bread flour, plus extra for dusting

1 tsp extra virgin olive oil (optional)

Pinch of salt

3 tbsp warm water

1. Put everything into a bowl and mix together to form a dough. Turn it onto a work surface and knead for 5 minutes, until smooth and elastic. If the dough seems wet and sticky, dust with a bit more flour as you knead it until it behaves. Divide it in half and form each piece into a ball. Allow to rest for 5 minutes.

2. Dust the work surface and a rolling pin with a little extra flour. Using your palms, squash the balls into fat discs, then roll them out as thinly as you can, aiming to keep them roughly circular.

3. Put a dry non-stick frying pan over a high heat and get it good and hot. Cook the flatbreads in it, one at a time, until lightly coloured and starting to blister – about 30 seconds a side. If you are cooking on a gas hob or barbecue, you can flip-flop the flatbreads across the open flames a couple of times with a pair of tongs to get some extra colour and to impress your friends.

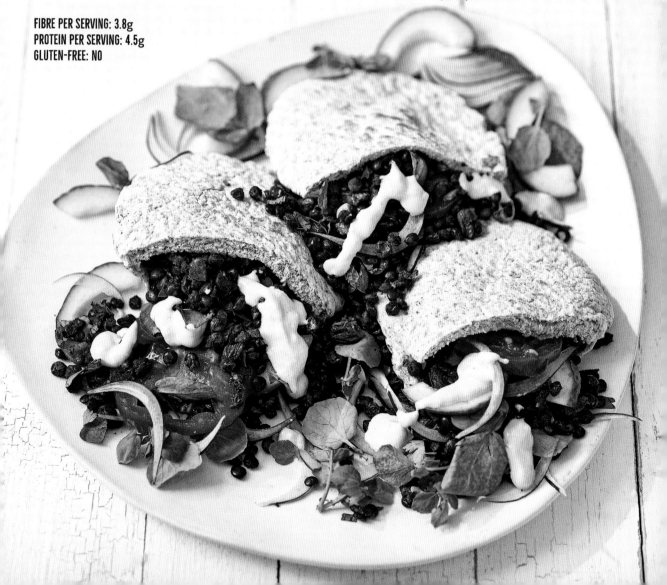

PLANT-POWERED STEW WITH BRAISED CHICKPEAS & COUSCOUS

There are 12 different plants in this dish, but the real star is the aubergine. Baking it whole allows the inside to soften beautifully while the skin blisters in the heat of the oven. Enjoy.

Serves 2
Prep & cook: 45 minutes

PLANT SCORE: 12
FIBRE PER SERVING: 17g
PROTEIN PER SERVING: 20g
GLUTEN-FREE: YES, IF YOU OMIT THE COUSCOUS

1 large aubergine

1 tbsp extra virgin olive oil (optional)

1 red onion, sliced

1 red pepper, deseeded and sliced

1 garlic clove, finely chopped

50g (½ cup) green olives, roughly chopped

1 tsp ground cumin

1 tsp smoked paprika

1½ tbsp harissa

1 x 400g (14oz) can chopped tomatoes or passata

200ml (¾ cup) vegetable stock

100g (1 cup) baby spinach

1 lemon

Sea salt and freshly ground black pepper

FOR THE BRAISED CHICKPEAS

1 x 400g (14oz) can chickpeas

Pinch of saffron (optional)

½ cinnamon stick

60g (⅓ cup) wholegrain couscous

About 100ml (½ cup) boiling water

Handful of parsley, chopped

Few fresh mint leaves, chopped

1. Preheat the oven to 220°C/Fan 180°C/400°F/Gas 8. Put the aubergine on a baking tray and place in the oven for 30 minutes, turning once or twice, until it is soft and collapsing and the skin is blistered. Pinch it with a pair of tongs to check. Set aside to cool slightly.

2. Warm the olive oil (if using) or a few tablespoons water in a large saucepan, then add the onion and red pepper. Fry over a medium heat for 15 minutes, until soft and starting to colour. Add a dash more water if the mixture looks like catching.

3. Meanwhile, tip the chickpeas and their liquid into a large saucepan. Add the saffron (if using) and cinnamon and bring to a simmer. Cook gently for 20 minutes, until the chickpeas are very soft and starting to break down.

4. When the onion mixture is ready, stir in the garlic, olives, cumin, paprika and harissa. Fry for 1 minute before adding the tomatoes and stock. Bring to a simmer and cook for 10 minutes or so.

5. When the chickpeas are ready, stir in the couscous and add the boiling water, just enough to cover everything. Cover the pan and set aside for 5–10 minutes, until the couscous has plumped up and become tender.

6. When the aubergines are cool enough to handle, peel away and discard the burnt skin; don't be too fussy, the odd fleck adds a bit of smokiness. Roughly chop the flesh and stir it into the stew along with the spinach. Taste and adjust the seasoning with salt, pepper and a squeeze or two of lemon juice.

7. Use a fork to fluff up the couscous and chickpeas. Stir in the parsley and mint just before serving with the stew.

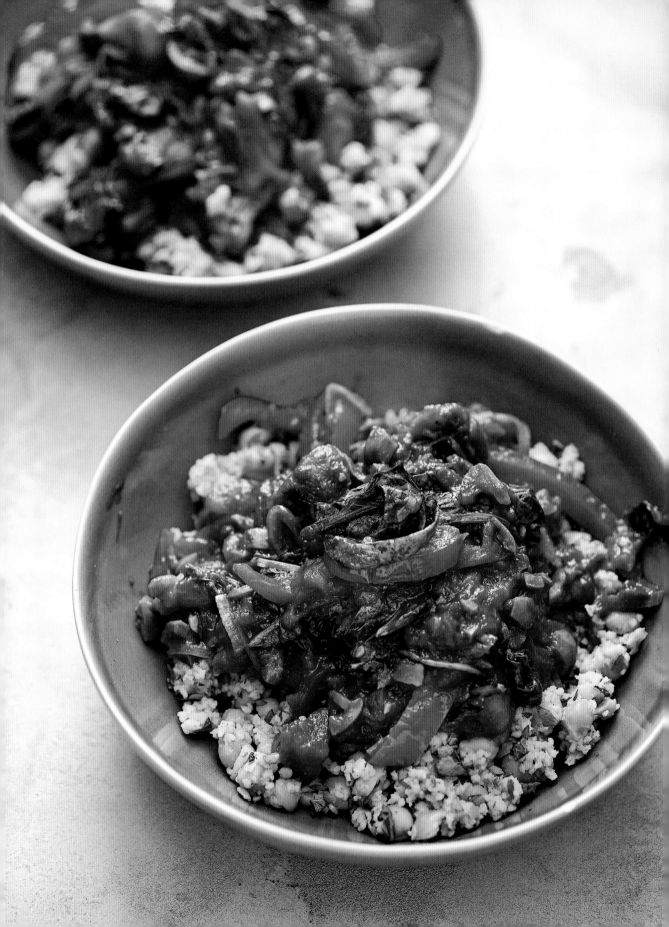

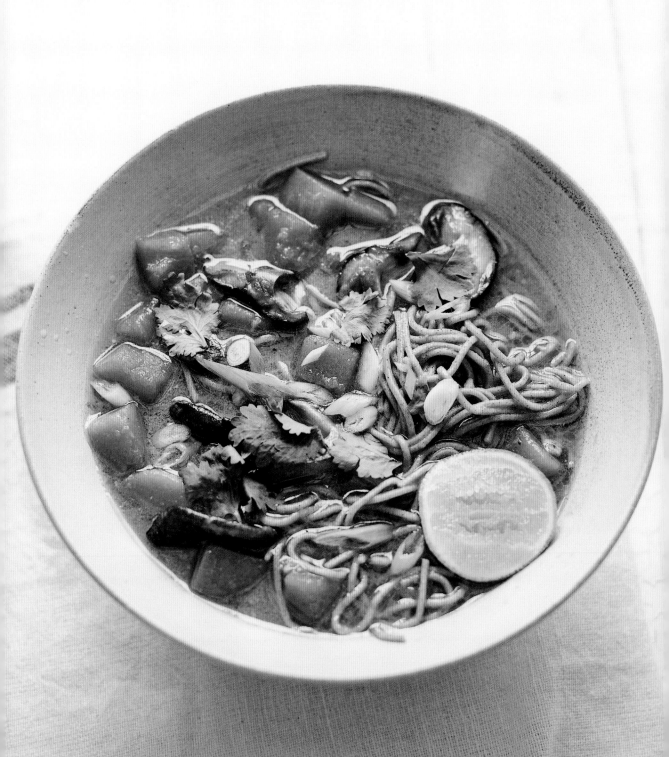

SQUASH & LEMONGRASS NOODLE BROTH

A hearty bowl of noodles is always a winner. If you'd like it even heartier, you can add about 200g (¾ cup) diced firm tofu to the pan too. The veg can be switched up, depending on the time of year – peas, radishes, pak choi and asparagus would work well in late spring, and could all be added in the final 5 minutes of cooking.

Serves 2
Cook & prep 40 minutes

PLANT SCORE: 8
FIBRE PER SERVING: 22g
PROTEIN PER SERVING: 24g
GLUTEN-FREE: YES, IF USING TAMARI RATHER THAN SOY SAUCE

100g (1½ cups) Portobello or shiitake mushrooms, thinly sliced

300g (2 cups) butternut squash, chopped into 1cm (½ inch) dice

1 garlic clove, finely chopped

2cm (¾ inch) fresh root ginger, finely grated

1 red chilli, deseeded and roughly chopped

1 tsp ground turmeric

1 tsp ground coriander

200ml (¾ cup) half-fat coconut milk

450ml (scant 2 cups) vegetable stock

2 tbsp tamari or soy sauce

2 lemongrass sticks, dry outer leaves discarded

100g (4oz) buckwheat noodles

2 spring onions, thinly sliced

Small handful of fresh coriander, roughly chopped

1 lime

1. Put the kettle on to boil, ready for step 5.

2. Warm 2 tablespoons water in a deep saucepan. Add the mushrooms and cook over a medium heat for 5 minutes, until starting to soften and colour.

3. Add the squash and cook for 2 minutes, before adding the garlic, ginger, chilli, turmeric and ground coriander. Fry for 30 seconds, making sure the spices don't stick and burn – add a dash of water if they look like doing so. Pour in the coconut milk, stock and tamari and bring to a gentle simmer.

4. Using a rolling pin, bash the root end of each lemongrass stick, then place in the pan to infuse their flavour. Simmer the broth gently for about 20 minutes, until the squash is tender.

5. Meanwhile, place the noodles in a large bowl and cover them with boiling water from the kettle. Set aside to soften; this should take about 5 minutes, depending on what brand you use. Cool immediately in cold water and drain well.

6. When the squash is ready, remove the lemongrass from the pan and stir in the spring onions, fresh coriander and a generous squeeze of lime. Taste and adjust the seasoning as you see fit.

7. Divide the cold noodles between 2 generous bowls. Ladle the hot broth over them, making sure the veg is shared equally.

STUFFED PEPPERS WITH ARTICHOKES, FENNEL & FARRO

It's time to reinvent this veggie classic. This updated version pops with the flavours of fresh basil, briny capers, juicy olives and slow-cooked tomatoes. It also uses wholegrain farro, which is lighter than brown rice and has a delicious nutty flavour.

Serves 2
Prep & cook: 50 minutes

PLANT SCORE: 10
FIBRE PER SERVING: 15g
PROTEIN PER SERVING: 12g
GLUTEN-FREE: MAKE THIS RECIPE GLUTEN-FREE BY USING BROWN BASMATI RICE INSTEAD OF THE FARRO.

1 fennel bulb, cut into thin wedges

½ tbsp extra virgin olive oil, plus extra for drizzling if you wish

4 tomatoes

2 red peppers, halved and deseeded

2 garlic cloves, thinly sliced

40g (2 rounded tbsp) capers, roughly chopped

60g (½ cup) pitted black olives, roughly sliced

20g (1 cup) fresh basil, plus extra to garnish

150g (¾ cup) preserved artichoke hearts, sliced. When ready, cool in a sieve under cold running water. Set aside to drain.

80g (½ cup) wholegrain farro

1 garlic clove, finely chopped

1 bay leaf

125ml (½ cup) white wine

350ml (1½ cups) hot vegetable stock

Sea salt and freshly ground black pepper

1. Put the kettle on to boil. Preheat the oven to 180°C/Fan 160°C/350°F/Gas 4.

2. Place the fennel in a deep roasting tray with the olive oil, a dash of water and a pinch of salt. Mix well and place in the oven for 12 minutes, until lightly coloured.

3. Cut a small cross in the top of each tomato and place them in a heatproof bowl. Cover them with boiling water and let them sit for about 1 minute, until the skins begin to loosen. Lift them out with a slotted spoon and, when cool enough to handle, peel off and discard the skin. Cut each tomato in half. (The skinning isn't vital, but it's a nice touch.)

4. Place the pepper halves on a work surface and divide the garlic, capers and olives equally between them. Add some torn basil leaves, then top with 2 tomato halves, cut side down, so that they cover the filling. Drizzle with a little olive oil (if using).

5. Remove the fennel tray from the oven and throw in the artichokes, farro, garlic, bay leaf, wine and stock. Sit the peppers in the tray too and cover tightly with foil. Return to the oven for another 20 minutes. The farro will absorb some of the stock and plump up as it cooks.

6. Uncover the tray, then return it to the oven for a final 10 minutes so that the peppers can colour slightly. You can add a dash of water too if the farro looks a little dry; you want it to be tender and fairly loose. Taste and adjust the seasoning if needed.

7. Serve the farro, veg and sauce in shallow bowls, topped with the peppers and some freshly torn basil to finish.

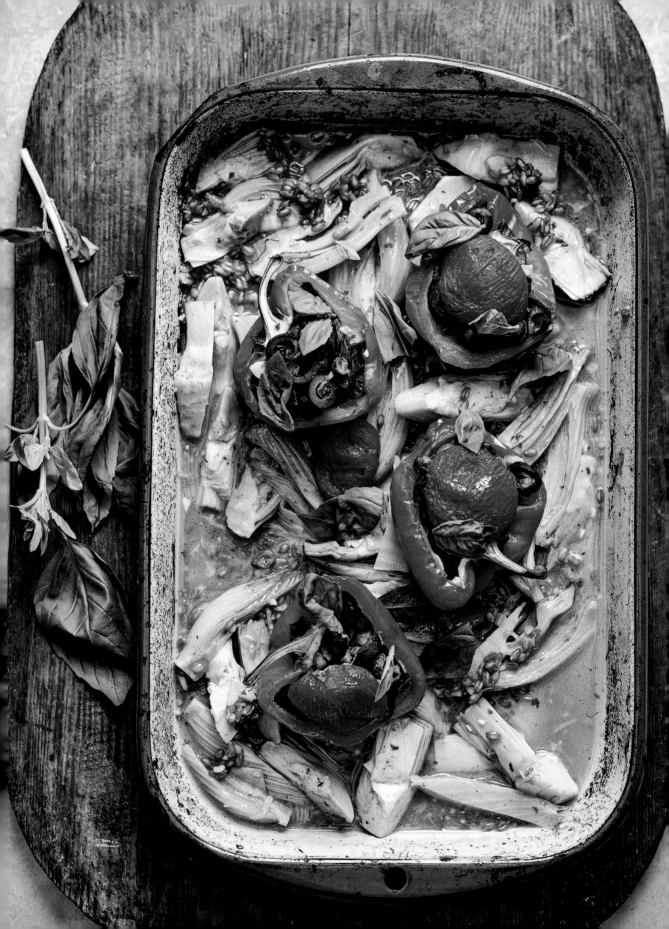

SUMMER VEG & WHITE BEAN PASTA

This dish is green, clean and fresh, lifted by the fresh herbs and lemon. The cannellini beans make it more substantial, while also bringing a comforting creaminess and a generous amount of protein per serving. To turn this into an autumn dish, use some grated squash and wild mushrooms instead of the asparagus and broad beans, and a garnish of thyme and hazelnuts rather than basil and pine nuts.

Serves 2
Prep & cook: 30 minutes

PLANT SCORE: 12
FIBRE PER SERVING: 22g
PROTEIN PER SERVING: 35g
GLUTEN-FREE: YES, IF USING GLUTEN-FREE PASTA

1 tbsp extra virgin olive oil (optional)

1 courgette, cut into 1cm (½ inch) dice

1 garlic clove, finely chopped

125ml (½ cup) white wine

1 x 400g (14oz) can cannellini beans, drained and rinsed

200ml (¾ cup) light vegetable stock

150g (1 generous cup) asparagus, trimmed and sliced into bite-sized pieces

100g (⅔ cup) podded fresh or frozen broad beans or edamame beans

80g (¾ cup) frozen peas

2 spring onions, thinly sliced

Zest and juice of ½ lemon

200g (2 cups) small wholemeal pasta shells

Sea salt and freshly ground black pepper

FOR THE GARNISH

20g (1 cup) fresh basil

6 fresh mint leaves

30g (¼ cup) toasted pine nuts

1 tbsp capers

1. Put a pan of water on to boil for the pasta.

2. Warm the oil (if using) or a few tablespoons water in a large saucepan. Add the courgette and cook gently over a medium-low heat for 10 minutes, until starting to soften.

3. Meanwhile, roughly chop the garnish ingredients together with half the lemon zest from the main list. Set aside until needed.

4. Add the garlic to the courgette pan and cook for 2 more minutes, before adding the wine. Let it bubble and reduce by half.

5. Put the pasta on to cook in boiling water. At the same time, add the cannellini beans and stock to the courgette pan. Bring to a gentle simmer, then cover and cook for 8 minutes, until the beans are starting to collapse.

6. Add the asparagus, broad beans, peas and spring onions to the courgette mixture. Cook for 5 minutes, until everything is tender. Taste and tweak the seasoning with salt, pepper and a dash or 2 of lemon juice, if needed. If it seems too thick add a dash of the pasta cooking water too.

7. Drain the pasta, tip it into the veg pan and stir together. Divide it between 2 bowls and garnish with the chopped herb mixture.

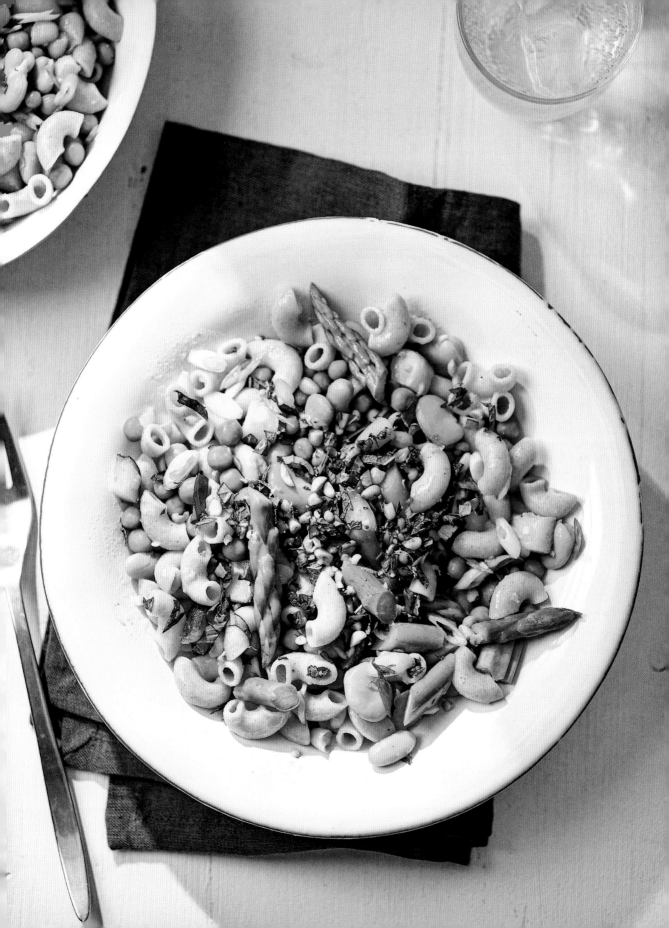

TEMPEH MISO STIR-FRY

Miso is one of my favourite fermented foods. Think of it as concentrated savouriness. For a darker, more wintry sauce you can use brown rice miso instead of white. Remember that stir-fries cook quickly, so make sure you have all the ingredients prepared before you start cooking. If you are cooking oil-free, use a really good non-stick pan and see the tips on frying without oil on page 60.

Serves 2
Prep & cook: 30 minutes

PLANT SCORE: 12
FIBRE PER SERVING: 14g
PROTEIN PER SERVING: 31g
GLUTEN-FREE: YES, IF USING TAMARI RATHER THAN SOY SAUCE

150g (6oz) buckwheat or brown rice noodles

1 tbsp extra virgin olive oil (optional)

100g (4oz) tempeh, cut into 1 cm (½ inch) pieces

125g (1½ cups) tenderstem broccoli, sliced into 2cm (¾ inch) pieces

125g (1¾ cups) shiitake mushrooms, sliced or torn

2 spring onions, finely sliced

1 baby pak choi, thinly shredded

15g (½ cup) sprouted seeds or beans, ideally, kale, broccoli, alfalfa or mung

Small handful of fresh coriander, finely chopped

½ tbsp sesame seeds

MISO SAUCE

1½ tbsp sweet white miso

½ tbsp brown rice vinegar

½ tbsp tamari or soy sauce

1 tsp finely grated fresh root ginger

1 garlic clove, finely chopped

1 lime

1. Cook the noodles in a pan of boiling water according to the packet instructions. Drain and cool straight away under cold running water. Drain thoroughly and set aside.

2. Put all the sauce ingredients, apart from the lime, into a small bowl, add 2 tablespoons water and mix. Tweak the taste to your liking with a squeeze or two of lime juice.

3. Heat ½ tablespoon of the oil (if using) in a large non-stick frying pan or wok. Throw in the tempeh and stir-fry for a couple of minutes, until golden. (Alternatively, if your non-stick pan is good, you should be able to colour the tempeh without any oil; just keep it moving and take care not to let it burn.) Transfer to a plate until needed.

4. Return the pan to the heat and add another ½ tablespoon oil (if using) or 2 tablespoons water. Throw in the broccoli and mushrooms and stir-fry on a high heat for 2 minutes. Add the spring onions and pak choi for a final minute. If at any point things look like catching and burning, add a dash of water.

5. Add the sauce and noodles to the pan and toss everything together for 30 seconds to heat through.

6. Remove from the heat and toss through the sprouted seeds/beans.

7. Divide the stir-fry between 2 plates and garnish with the fresh coriander and sesame seeds.

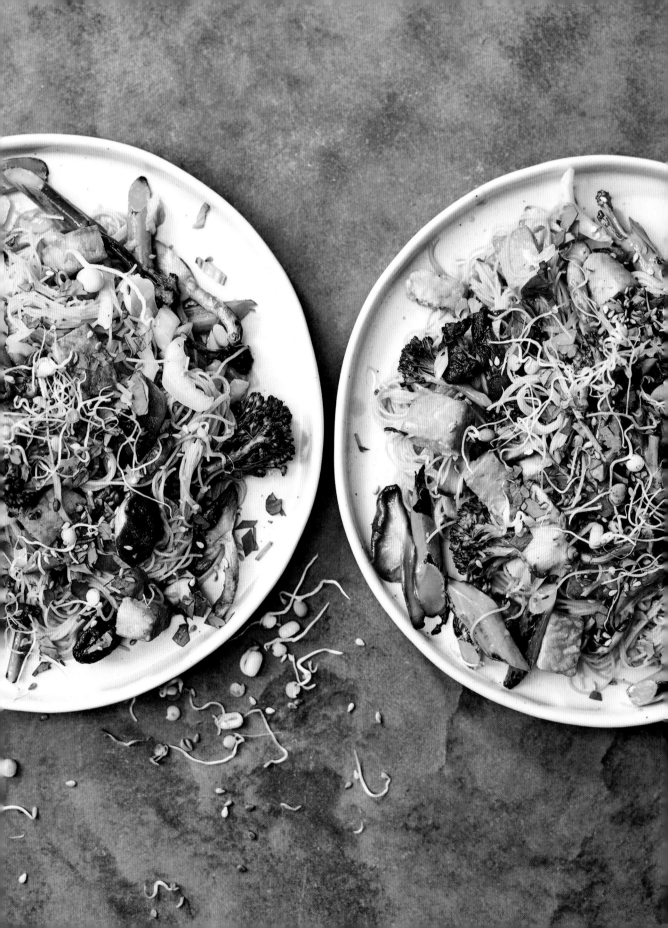

WINTER BARLEY STEW WITH IRISH STOUT & HERBY DUMPLINGS

With plenty of root veg and 23g of plant protein per bowl, this hearty stew really provides everything you need to fill up on a cold winter's day. Add the herby dumpling to increase the comfort!

Serves 2
Prep & cook: 45 minutes

PLANT SCORE: 11
FIBRE PER SERVING: 14g
PROTEIN PER SERVING: 23g
GLUTEN-FREE: NO

½ tbsp extra virgin olive oil (optional)

1 leek, finely sliced

1 carrot, cut into 1cm (½ inch) dice

2 celery sticks, diced

100g (1½ cups) chestnut mushrooms, quartered

¼ swede, peeled and cut into 1cm (½ inch) dice

1 potato, cut into 1cm (½ inch) dice

80g (⅓ cup) pearl barley

1 garlic clove, finely chopped

1 tsp fresh thyme leaves

1 bay leaf

1 tbsp tomato purée

1 tbsp tamari or soy sauce

1 tbsp wholemeal flour

330ml (1⅓ cups) dark stout

400ml (1¾ cups) vegetable stock

100g (4 cups) black kale, roughly chopped

Sea salt and freshly ground black pepper

FOR THE HERBY DUMPLINGS

60g (⅓ cup + 1 tbsp) wholemeal self-raising flour

Pinch of salt

½ tsp fresh thyme leaves

1 tbsp nutritional yeast flakes

½ tbsp extra virgin olive oil (optional)

40ml (scant 3 tbsp) almond milk or water

1. Preheat the oven to 180°C/Fan 160°C/350°F/Gas 4.

2. Warm the olive oil (if using) or a few tablespoons water in a large saucepan or flameproof casserole dish. Add the leek, carrot and celery and cook over a low heat for 10 minutes, until starting to soften. Add a dash of water if they look like catching at any point.

3. Increase the heat to medium and throw in the mushrooms. Cook for 5 minutes, until they start to darken.

4. Add the swede, potato, barley, garlic, thyme and bay, and cook for a further 5 minutes.

5. Stir in the tomato purée, tamari and flour and cook for 2 minutes, stirring constantly to avoid the flour sticking and burning.

6. Pour in the stout and stock, bring to a simmer and season lightly with salt and pepper. Cover and transfer to the oven for 25 minutes.

7. To make the dumplings, put the flour, salt, thyme and yeast flakes into a bowl and stir together. Gently mix in the olive oil (if using) and milk just until a dough forms. Make sure you don't overmix. If it seems too dry, add a dash more milk; if too sticky, add a touch more flour. Divide the dough into 4 equal pieces and gently roll each one into a ball.

8. Remove the stew from the oven, stir in the kale, then return to the oven for another 15 minutes, until the kale is dark and wilted.

9. Sit the dumplings on top of the stew, pushing them down so they are half-submerged. Cook for 25 more minutes, until the dumplings are plumped up and cooked through.

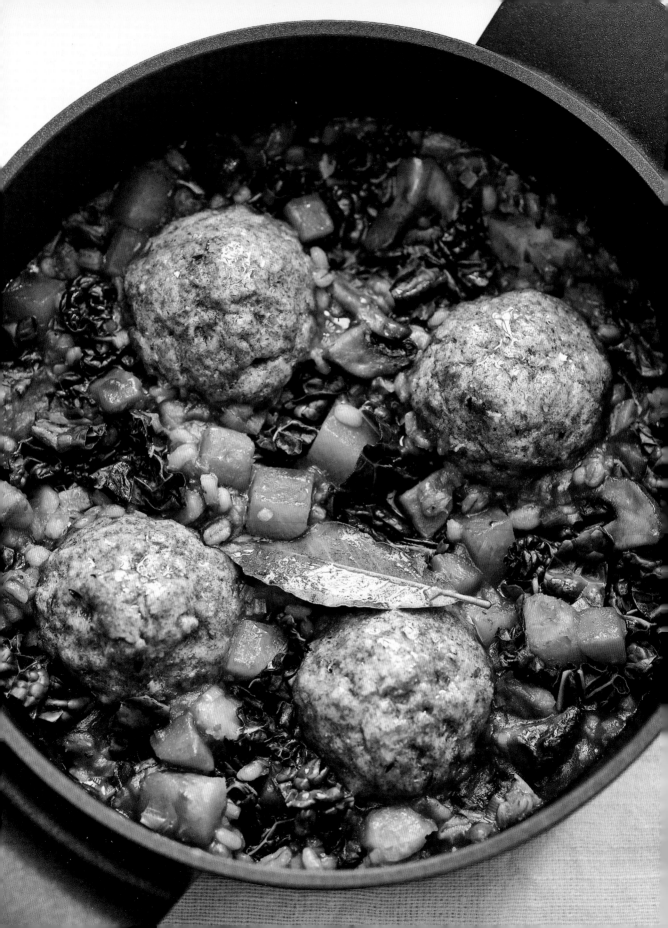

STICKY TOFU, COURGETTES, GREENS & KIMCHI

The sweet stickiness of the tofu comes from the marinade, as it quickly reduces to a glossy sauce in the hot pan. A generous amount of kimchi adds probiotic benefits and some extra flavour to this deceptively simple dish.

Serves 2
Prep & cook: 35 minutes

PLANT SCORE: 8
FIBRE PER SERVING: 9.4g
PROTEIN PER SERVING: 27g
GLUTEN-FREE: YES, IF USING TAMARI RATHER THAN SOY SAUCE

150g (¾ cup) brown rice

200g (7 oz) firm or extra-firm tofu, preferably smoked

2 courgettes, cut into 1cm (½ inch) slices

1 small pak choi, roughly shredded

1 tbsp sesame seeds

1 lime

100g (¾ cup) kimchi

FOR THE MARINADE

1 garlic clove, finely chopped

½ tbsp finely chopped ginger

1 tbsp rice vinegar

2 tbsp tamari or soy sauce

1 tbsp maple syrup

1. Put a kettle on to boil. Meanwhile, rinse the rice in a sieve under cold running water. Tip it into a saucepan, cover with plenty of boiling water, stir once and simmer for 25–30 minutes, until tender. (Remember that cooked brown rice still has a little chewiness to it.)

2. While the rice cooks, cut the tofu into 6 equal pieces and place in a bowl with all the marinade ingredients. Set aside until needed.

3. Put a pan of water on to boil, or get a steamer ready for the veg.

4. About 5 minutes before the rice is ready put a large non-stick frying pan over a medium-high heat. Scrape as much of the marinade off the tofu slices as you can. Place them flat in the pan and fry for about 2 minutes on each side, until starting to catch and colour. Tip the marinade into the pan and let it bubble for a minute or so, until thick and sticky, turning the tofu in it to coat.

5. Boil or steam the courgettes and pak choi for 3 minutes, or until just tender. Drain and toss with the sesame seeds and a squeeze of lime juice.

6. Divide the rice between 2 shallow bowls, sit the greens and kimchi alongside it and top with the sticky tofu.

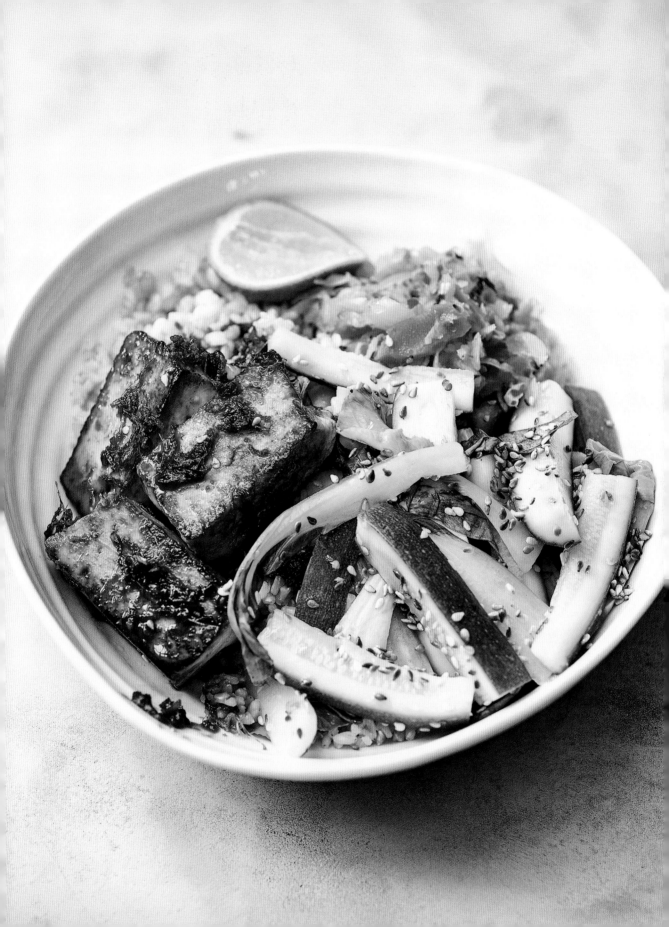

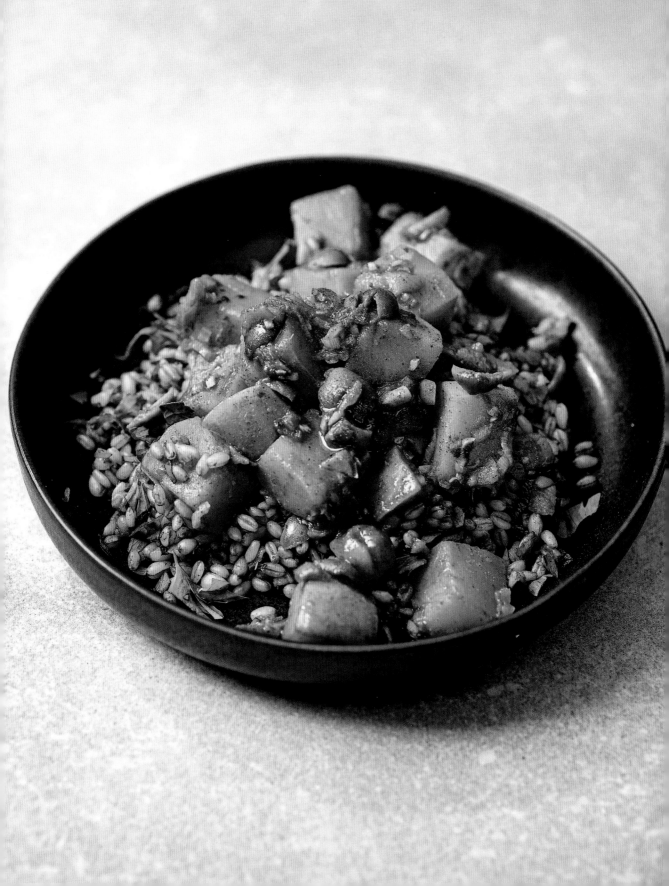

SQUASH & OLIVE TAGINE WITH FREEKEH

Freekeh are roasted green grains, full of wholegrain goodness and a light smoky taste. Try to find cracked freekeh, as its much faster to cook. If you can't get hold of freekeh, use bulgur wheat and follow the cooking instructions on the packet. Preserved lemons, a traditional North African ingredient, add their unique and intense flavour to this easy tagine, and are now stocked in many supermarkets.

Serves 2
Prep & cook: 40 minutes

PLANT SCORE: 10
FIBRE PER SERVING: 18g
PROTEIN PER SERVING: 15g
GLUTEN-FREE: YES, IF USING WHOLEGRAIN RICE INSTEAD OF FREEKEH; IN THIS CASE, INCREASE THE COOKING TIME TO 30 MINUTES

400ml (1¾ cups) vegetable stock

1 red onion, finely sliced

2 garlic cloves, finely chopped

1 tsp ground coriander

1 tsp ground cumin

1 tsp ground ginger

½ tsp smoked paprika

½ tsp ground cinnamon

600g (4 cups) butternut squash, cut into 2cm (¾ inch) dice

60g (½ cup) green olives, sliced

40g (⅓ cup) dried apricots, roughly chopped

½ preserved lemon or 1 fresh lemon

120g (¾ cup) cracked freekeh

400ml (1¾ cups) boiling water

1 tbsp harissa

Small handful of parsley, finely chopped

6 fresh mint leaves, finely chopped

1. Pour the stock into a large saucepan, add the onion, garlic and spices and bring to a gentle simmer.

2. Add the squash, olives and apricots to the pan. If using preserved lemon, scrape away and discard the soft interior, then finely chop the skin and add it to the pan. If using a fresh lemon, cut 2 long strips of zest with a vegetable peeler and add them to the pan along with a big squeeze of lemon juice. Bring everything to a simmer, pop on a lid and cook gently for 25 minutes, or until the squash is completely soft.

3. Meanwhile, place the freekeh in another large saucepan, add the boiling water and bring to a simmer. Cook for about 20 minutes, until the freekeh is tender. Drain off any excess liquid, then stir in the harissa, parsley and mint.

4. Divide the freekeh between shallow bowls and spoon the tagine over the top.

ROASTING TRAY RATATOUILLE GRATIN

This simple gratin puts beans, greens and wholegrains on your plate. Make sure to cover the tray nice and tightly with foil so that the veg cook perfectly without scorching.

Serves 2
Prep & cook: 1 hour

PLANT SCORE: 13
FIBRE PER SERVING: 24g
PROTEIN PER SERVING: 24g
GLUTEN-FREE: YES, IF USING GLUTEN-FREE BREAD

1 small aubergine, cut into 2cm (¾ inch) pieces

1 courgette, cut into 2cm (¾ inch) pieces

300g (2 cups) cherry tomatoes, halved

1 red onion, sliced

1 red pepper, deseeded and cut into 2cm (¾ inch) pieces

1 yellow pepper, deseeded and cut into 2cm (¾ inch) pieces

1 tbsp extra virgin olive oil (optional)

2 tbsp balsamic vinegar

150g (about 4 slices) stale wholemeal bread, crusts removed

½ tbsp fresh oregano or thyme leaves.

Zest of 1 lemon

Small handful of fresh basil leaves

1 x 400g (14oz) can borlotti beans, drained and rinsed

2 garlic cloves, finely chopped

Sea salt and freshly ground black pepper

1. Preheat the oven to 200ºC/Fan 180ºC/400ºF/Gas 6.

2. Put the aubergine, courgette, tomatoes, onion and peppers into a large roasting tray. Add the olive oil (if using), the vinegar and 3 tablespoons water. Season lightly with salt and pepper and cover tightly with foil. Transfer to the oven and bake for 35 minutes, removing the foil for the final 10 minutes so the veg can get a bit of colour.

3. Meanwhile, put the bread in a food processor or blender, add the oregano, lemon zest and a few twists of black pepper and pulse into coarse breadcrumbs.

4. Remove the tray from the oven and reduce the heat to 180ºC/Fan 160ºC/350ºF/Gas 4. Tear the basil and stir it into the vegetables, along with the beans and garlic. Arrange the breadcrumbs over the top in an even layer. Return the tray to the oven and cook for further 15–20 minutes, until the top is golden and crisp.

5. Serve with some freshly steamed greens on the side.

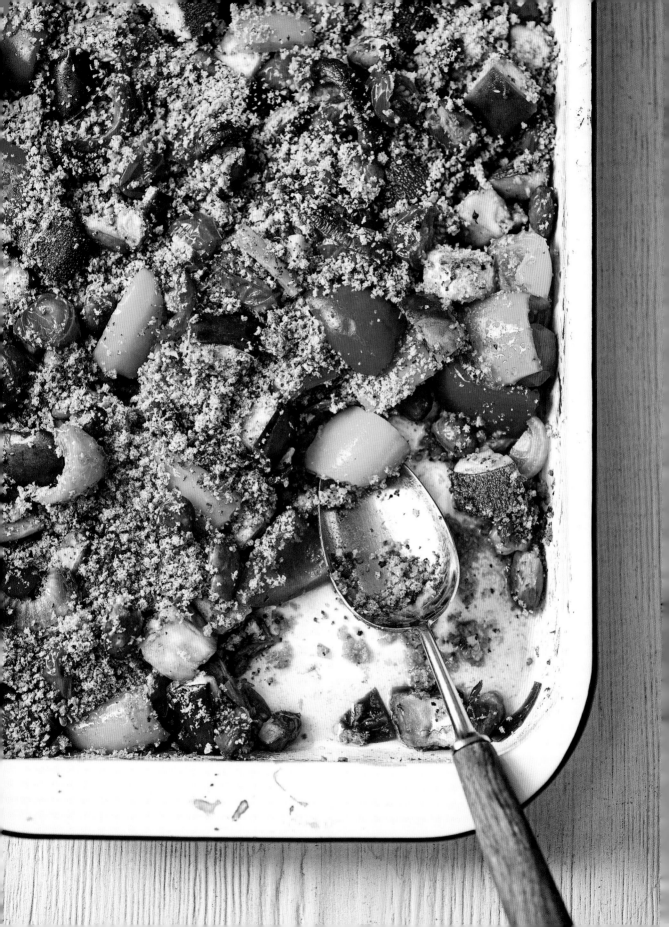

SWEET POTATO MASSAMAN CURRY

The complex flavours of this dish are provided by an array of aromatic spices. You can control the heat by using as little or as much curry paste as you like.

Serves 2
Prep & cook: 40 minutes

PLANT SCORE: 9
FIBRE PER SERVING: 15g
PROTEIN PER SERVING: 23g
GLUTEN-FREE: YES

150g (¾ cup) brown basmati rice

3 spring onions, finely sliced

300g (11oz) or about 2 sweet potatoes, cut into 2cm (¾ inch) dice

1 x 400g (14oz) can chickpeas, drained and rinsed

20g (1 rounded tbsp) salted peanuts, coarsely chopped

2–3 tbsp red Thai curry paste, depending on what heat you like

4 cardamom pods

1 star anise

1 tsp ground cumin

½ tsp ground turmeric

½ cinnamon stick

200ml (¾ cup) half-fat coconut milk

500ml (2 cups) vegetable stock or water

80g (¾ cup) French beans, chopped into 2cm (¾ inch) pieces

Small handful of fresh coriander

1 lime

Sea salt

1. Rinse the rice in a sieve under cold running water. Tip it into a medium saucepan and cover with plenty of boiling water. Stir once and simmer for 25–30 minutes, until tender, but still slightly chewy.

2. Put the onions, sweet potato, chickpeas, peanuts, curry paste and spices into a large saucepan. Pour in the coconut milk and stock and bring to a gentle simmer. Cook for 25 minutes, until the potatoes are soft, adding the French beans halfway through the cooking time.

3. When ready, stir in half the coriander and a good squeeze of lime juice. Taste and tweak to your liking with lime juice and salt.

4. Serve the curry with the rice and garnish with the remaining coriander. You can remove the cinnamon stick, star anise and cardamom pods before serving if you like, or just eat around them.

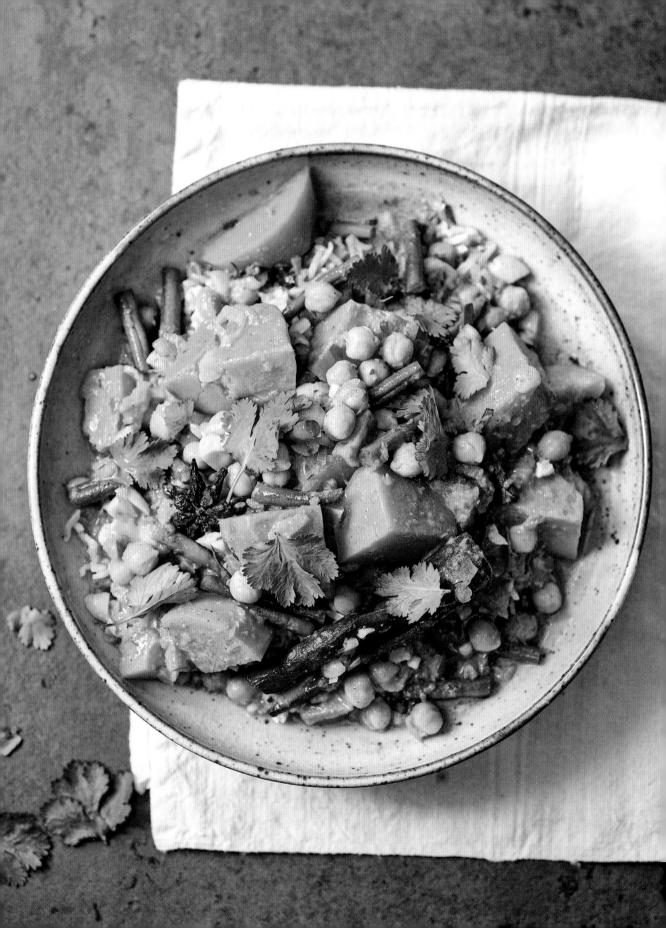

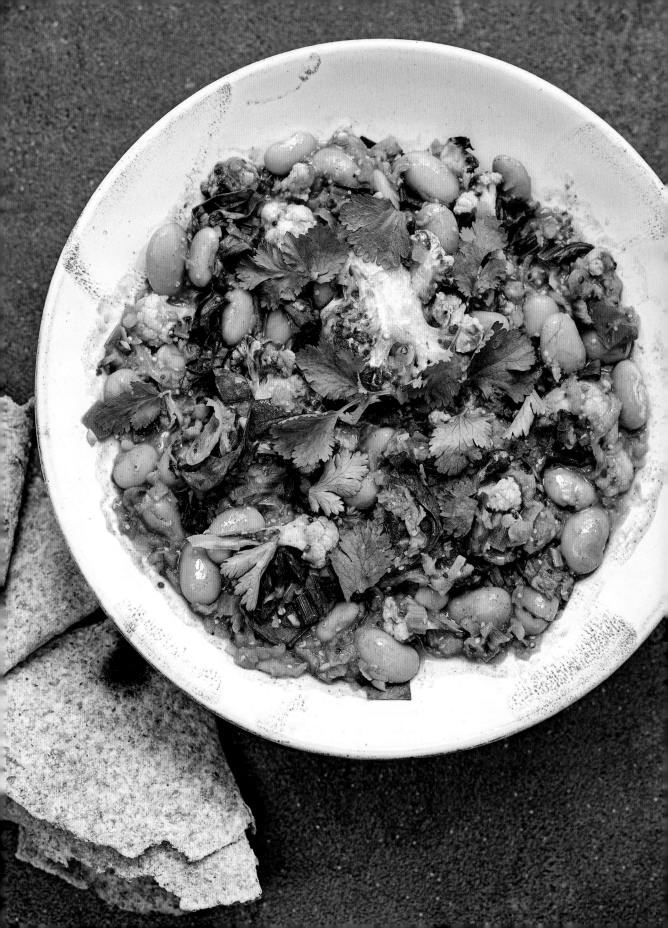

CAULIFLOWER, BUTTER BEAN & CHARD DAHL

You can add the cauliflower straight into the dahl without frying it first, but a few minutes in the pan will add extra colour and really deepen the flavour. If you don't have chard, use spinach instead. You don't need to remove the stalks from the spinach – just add the leaves whole at the very end and stir them through to wilt down in the heat of the dish.

Serves 2
Prep & cook: 45 minutes

PLANT SCORE: 10
FIBRE PER SERVING: 19g
PROTEIN PER SERVING: 29g
GLUTEN-FREE: YES, IF SERVED WITH RICE OR GLUTEN-FREE FLATBREADS

100g (4oz) chard, stalks and leaves separated

1 red onion, finely sliced

150g (¾ cup) tomatoes, roughly chopped

80g (¾ cup) red lentils, rinsed

2 garlic cloves, finely chopped

1 tbsp finely grated fresh root ginger

1 red chilli, deseeded and finely chopped

1 tsp ground turmeric

1 tsp ground cumin

1 tsp garam masala

1 x 400g (14oz) can butter beans, drained and rinsed

500ml (2 cups) vegetable stock

½ tbsp extra virgin olive oil (optional)

½ cauliflower, cut into 1cm (½ inch) slices

1 tbsp wholegrain mustard

1 lemon

Sea salt and freshly ground black pepper

Small handful of fresh coriander, to garnish

Brown rice or wholemeal flatbreads, to serve

1. Finely dice the chard stalks and throw them into a large saucepan with the onion, tomatoes and 3 tablespoons water. Cook gently for 10 minutes, until starting to soften. Add a dash more water if they look like catching.

2. Add the lentils, garlic, ginger, chilli and spices. Cook for 2 more minutes before adding the butter beans and stock. Season lightly with salt and pepper and bring to a gentle simmer. Cook for 25–30 minutes, stirring frequently, until the lentils are completely soft. Top up with a dash of extra water if it looks too thick.

3. Meanwhile, warm the olive oil or a tablespoon water in a large non-stick frying pan. Fry the cauliflower over a medium heat for 2–3 minutes on each side, until golden brown. Add to the dahl along with the mustard for the final 10 minutes of cooking time.

4. When ready, finely shred the chard leaves and stir them into the dahl until wilted; this will take only a couple of minutes. Finish with a good squeeze of lemon juice. Taste and adjust the seasoning to your liking.

5. Serve the dahl alongside rice or flatbreads and garnish with the fresh coriander.

CAJUN BEANS & GREENS

A simple bean stew with flavours from the southern United States: the smoky paprika, soft-cooked rice and corn on the cob make a perfect combination.

Serves 2
Prep & cook: 1 hour

PLANT SCORE: 10
FIBRE PER SERVING: 10g
PROTEIN PER SERVING: 21g
GLUTEN-FREE: YES

1 tbsp extra virgin olive oil (optional)

1 celery stick, diced

1 green pepper, diced

60g (½ cup) French beans, finely sliced

2 garlic cloves, finely chopped

1 tsp fresh thyme leaves

1 tsp smoked paprika

½ tsp ground cumin

1 bay leaf

1 x 400g (14oz) can kidney beans, drained and rinsed

80g (½ cup) brown rice, rinsed

200g (1 generous cup) tomatoes, roughly chopped, or ½ can chopped tomatoes)

500ml (2 cups) vegetable stock

Cayenne pepper, to taste

2 sweetcorn cobs, husks removed

3 spring onions

100g (1 generous cup) baby spinach

1 lime, cut into wedges

Sea salt and freshly ground black pepper

1. Warm the olive oil (if using) or 3 tablespoons water in a large saucepan. Add the celery and green pepper and cook gently for 10 minutes, until starting to soften. Add a dash more water if they look like drying out at any point.

2. Add the French beans, garlic, thyme, paprika, cumin and bay leaf, and cook for 2 more minutes, stirring to make sure the spices don't stick. Tip in the kidney beans, rice, tomatoes and stock. Bring to a simmer and add cayenne pepper to taste. Season with plenty of black pepper and a little salt if needed. Cook gently for 30 minutes, or until the rice is cooked.

3. When the rice is ready, cook the corn in a pan of boiling water for 8 minutes, until tender.

4. Stir the spring onions and spinach into the stew. When the spinach has wilted, add a squeeze of lime juice. Taste and tweak the seasoning to your liking with more cayenne pepper and lime. Set aside until the corn is ready.

5. Serve the stew in deep bowls with the corn on the side. The corn will benefit from some black pepper and a little rub with a lime wedge.

SPANISH RICE WITH FENNEL, TOMATO & OLIVES

This plant-powered paella includes all the flavours of the original dish with the added benefits of wholegrain rice. Including a pinch of saffron is a nice authentic touch, but if you don't have any, a pinch of ground turmeric will add the same golden colour.

Serves 2
Prep & cook: 1 hour

PLANT SCORE: 11
FIBRE PER SERVING: 14g
PROTEIN PER SERVING: 18g
GLUTEN-FREE: YES

200g (generous cup) brown basmati rice

1 red onion, sliced

1 fennel bulb, trimmed and sliced

400g (2⅔ cups) cherry tomatoes, halved

1 tbsp extra virgin olive oil (optional)

50g (½ cup) green olives, sliced

100ml (½ cup) white wine

2 garlic cloves, finely chopped

Pinch of saffron (optional)

½ tsp ground fennel seeds

½ tsp ground cumin

1 tsp smoked paprika

Pinch of dried chilli flakes

600ml (2½ cups) boiling vegetable stock

50g (⅓ cup) frozen peas

150g (1½ cups) baby spinach

Sea salt and freshly ground black pepper

TO SERVE

30g (⅓ cup) flaked and toasted almonds (optional)

1 lemon, cut into wedges

1. Preheat the oven to 200°C/Fan 180°C/400°F/Gas 6. Place the rice in a bowl, cover it with cold water and set aside to soak until needed.

2. Place the onion, fennel and tomatoes into a large shallow casserole dish or roasting tray with the olive oil (if using) and 3 tablespoons water. Season lightly with salt and pepper, then transfer to the oven for 30 minutes, until everything has softened and started to colour at the edges. You might want to stir it once halfway through to get an even cook.

3. Drain and rinse the rice. Remove the pan from the oven and add the rice, olives, wine, garlic and spices. Stir everything to combine, then pour in the stock. Cover the pan with a lid or foil and return to the oven for 20–25 minutes, until the rice is cooked and plump.

4. Remove from the oven and stir in the peas and spinach. Cover the pan again and leave for a few minutes, until the spinach has wilted and the peas are cooked.

5. Garnish with toasted almonds if you're feeling fancy, and serve with the lemon wedges for squeezing over the top.

WINTER PILAF

Fragrant rice with some winter veg, nuts and fragrant spicing. Perfect!
Wild rice, available in most supermarkets, is a delicious wholegrain with a
higher protein content than other rice varieties.

Serves 2
Prep & cook: 50 minutes

PLANT SCORE: 12
FIBRE PER SERVING: 18g
PROTEIN PER SERVING: 23g
GLUTEN-FREE: YES

700ml (3 cups) vegetable stock

1 orange

6 cardamom pods

1 cinnamon stick

1 tsp ground cumin

150g (scant 1 cup) wild rice, rinsed

1 tbsp extra virgin olive oil (optional)

1 leek, finely diced

1 celery stick, finely diced

1 parsnip or ½ head of celeriac, cut into 1cm (½ inch) dice

½ small cauliflower, cut into small florets

2 garlic cloves, finely chopped

1 tsp finely chopped rosemary leaves

100g (4 cups) kale, stalks removed and roughly chopped

2 tbsp walnuts, roughly chopped

2 tbsp pumpkin seeds, roughly chopped

30g (3½ tbsp) dried cranberries, apricots or raisins, roughly chopped

Sea salt and freshly ground black pepper

1. Put the stock in a large saucepan and bring it to a simmer. Pare 4 long strips of zest from the orange and throw them into the stock. Add the cardamom pods, cinnamon stick and cumin, then pour in the rice. Return to a gentle simmer, cover loosely and simmer for about 45 minutes, until the rice is tender but still has a chewy bite. Keep an eye on the pan, adding a little more water if and when needed.

2. Meanwhile, warm the olive oil (if using) or 3 tablespoons water in another large saucepan. Add the leek, celery and parsnip and cook over a gentle heat for 10 minutes, until starting to soften. Add a dash more water if they look like drying out or catching at any point.

3. Add the cauliflower, garlic and rosemary with about 4 tablespoons water. Continue cooking gently for 6–8 minutes, then stir in the kale and cook for a final 4–5 minutes. If at any point it looks like drying out or burning, add a dash more water. Set aside until the rice is cooked.

4. Once the rice is ready, drain away any excess water. Tip the rice into the pan of veg. Add the nuts, seeds, dried fruit and a small squeeze of orange juice. Mix well, then taste and tweak the seasoning to your liking.

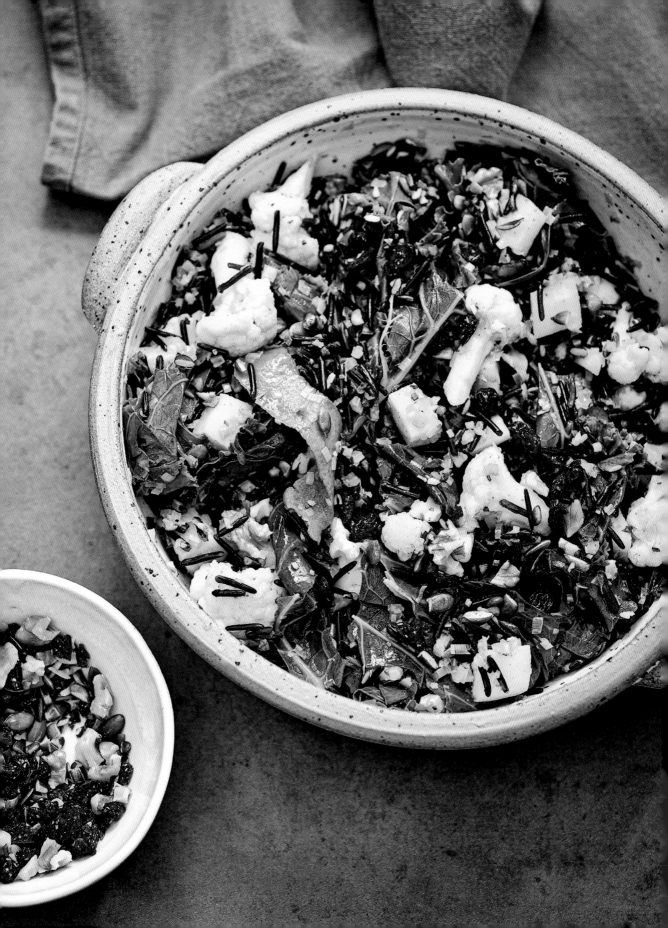

GOULASH HOTPOT

The deep flavours of the goulash bring this veggie hotpot to life. Make sure to use sweet paprika (not smoked) or the flavour will overwhelm the dish. You could also cook the goulash on its own and serve it up with mash, noodles or rice. Try serving with a dollop of sour cream on the side (see page 86).

Serves 2
Prep & cook: 1 hour

PLANT SCORE: 9
FIBRE PER SERVING: 27g
PROTEIN PER SERVING: 23g
GLUTEN-FREE: YES

1 onion, sliced

2 red peppers, deseeded and sliced

1 x 400g (14oz) can chickpeas, drained and rinsed

2 garlic cloves, finely chopped

2 tbsp sweet paprika

1 tbsp tomato purée

½ tsp caraway seeds

1 tsp dried oregano

1 x 400g (14oz) can chopped tomatoes

200ml (¾ cup) vegetable stock or water

Cayenne pepper

2 potatoes, thinly sliced

½ tbsp extra virgin olive oil (optional)

200g (3 cups) spring or summer greens, thinly sliced

1 lemon

Small handful of fresh dill, roughly chopped

Sea salt and freshly ground black pepper

1. Preheat the oven to 200°C/Fan 180°C/400°F/Gas 6.

2. Put the onion and peppers in a flameproof casserole dish with 3 tablespoons water. Place on the heat and cook gently for 10 minutes, until softened. Add a dash more water if the veg look like catching at any point.

3. Add the chickpeas, garlic, paprika, tomato purée, caraway and oregano. Cook for 2 minutes before adding the tomatoes, stock and a pinch of cayenne. Bring to a simmer and cook gently for 5 minutes. Taste and tweak the seasoning to your liking with pepper, salt and more cayenne.

4. Toss the sliced potatoes in a bowl with the oil, if using, and a pinch of salt. Arrange them in an overlapping pattern on top of the goulash. Transfer to the oven and bake for 40 minutes, or until the potatoes are cooked through and golden.

5. When the hotpot is ready, boil, steam or wilt the greens to your liking, and finish them with a squeeze of lemon juice and the chopped dill. Serve them alongside generous scoops of the hotpot.

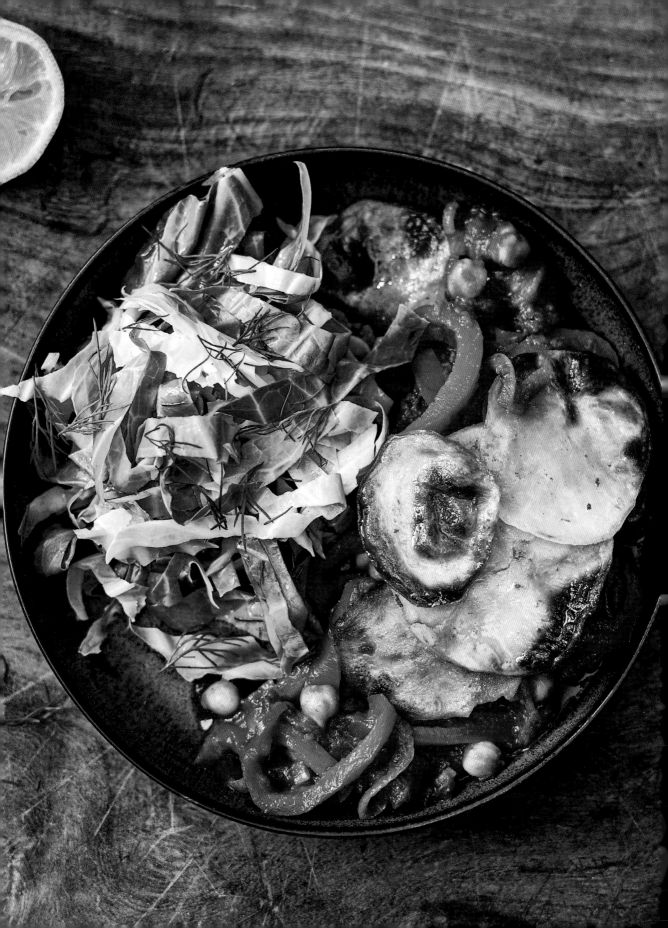

PAKORA BEAN BURGERS WITH RAITA & SWEET POTATO CHIPS

A classic bean burger meets an Indian pakora. Enjoy!

Serves 2
Prep & cook: 35 minutes

PLANT SCORE: 14
FIBRE PER SERVING: 26g
PROTEIN PER SERVING: 28g
GLUTEN-FREE: YES, IF USING GLUTEN-FREE BUNS AND CURRY PASTE

½ red onion, finely sliced

150g (1½ cups) coarsely grated carrot

2 large sweet potatoes

½ tbsp extra virgin olive oil (optional)

1 garlic clove, finely chopped

1½ tbsp curry paste of the heat you prefer, plus more to taste

1 x 400g (14oz) can black-eyed beans, drained and rinsed

3 tbsp chickpea (gram) flour, plus extra for tweaking

Small handful of fresh coriander, finely chopped

1 lemon

Sea salt and freshly ground black pepper

FOR THE RAITA

¼ cucumber

4 tbsp plain soya yogurt

4 fresh mint leaves, finely chopped

1 tsp black onion seeds (optional)

TO SERVE

2 wholegrain burger buns

1 tomato, sliced

Handful of salad leaves

1. Preheat the oven to 200ºC/Fan 180ºC/400ºF/Gas 6.

2. Place the onion and carrot in a large saucepan with 3 tablespoons water and cook over a gentle heat for 10 minutes, until starting to soften. Add a dash more water if they look like catching at any point, but you want the excess water to have been driven off by the heat.

3. Meanwhile, cut the sweet potatoes into long, thin fries. Lay them on a non-stick baking tray, drizzle with the olive oil (if using), and season lightly with salt and pepper. Turn and mix to coat.

4. Add the garlic and curry paste to the carrots and cook for 2 more minutes. Remove from the heat and tip in the beans, chickpea flour and coriander. Mix everything together aggressively – use a potato masher a few times if you like – to smash up the beans. Taste and tweak to your liking with a little lemon juice, salt and pepper. If the mix is a bit too wet to handle, mix in more chickpea flour until it just comes together. Form the mixture into two large flat burgers, about 2cm thick.

5. Heat a dry non-stick frying and fry the burgers for about 2 minutes on each side, until lightly coloured. Transfer to a clean baking tray.

6. Place the tray of sweet potatoes on the top shelf of the oven. Put the burgers on the shelf below. Cook the burgers for 10 minutes, until piping hot, and cook the fries for about 15 minutes, or until nicely coloured, turning once.

7. In the meantime, make the raita. Halve the cucumber lengthways and scoop out the seeds with the tip of a teaspoon. Coarsely grate the cucumber flesh and use your hands to squeeze out as much water as you can. Place the flesh in a bowl with the yogurt, mint and onion seeds and mix well.

8. When everything is ready, slice open the buns and sit some sliced tomato and salad leaves on the bottom halves. Add the burgers and a generous spoonful of raita, then top with the remaining bun halves. Serve alongside the fries.

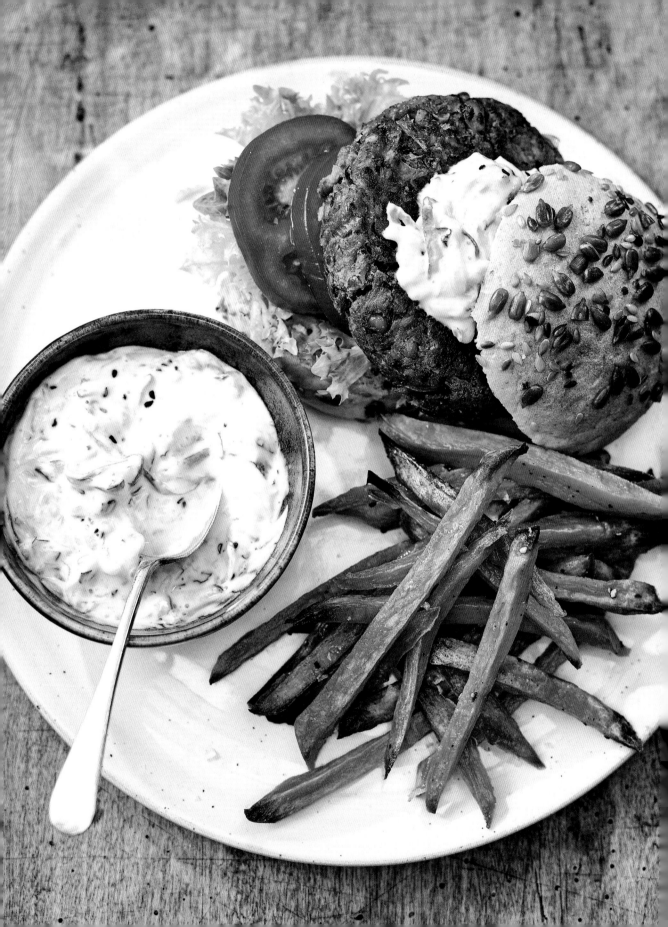

ONE-POT CHILLI BOWL

We've combined a classic bean chilli with the wholegrain goodness of quinoa to bring you a delicious protein-packed bowl.

Serves 2
Prep & cook: 35 minutes

PLANT SCORE: 9
FIBRE PER SERVING: 24g
PROTEIN PER SERVING: 24g
GLUTEN-FREE: YES

½ tbsp extra virgin olive oil (optional)

1 red onion, finely diced

1 red pepper, deseeded and diced

2 garlic cloves

1 red chilli, deseeded and finely chopped

½ tbsp ground cumin

1 tsp ground coriander

1 tsp dried oregano

½ tsp smoked paprika

½ tsp chilli powder, or to taste

¼ tsp ground cinnamon

125g (¾ cup) quinoa, rinsed

1 x 400g (14oz) can chopped tomatoes

1 x 400g (14oz) can kidney beans, drained and rinsed

400ml (1¾ cups) vegetable stock

Dried chilli flakes, for tweaking

1 avocado, sliced

Small handful of fresh coriander, finely chopped

Sea salt and freshly ground black pepper

Lime wedges, to serve

1. Warm the oil (if using) or 3 tablespoons water in a large saucepan. Add the onion and pepper and cook over a gentle heat for 10 minutes, until starting to soften. Add a dash more water if they look like catching at any point.

2. Add the garlic, red chilli, spices and quinoa. Cook for 2 minutes, stirring often to make sure nothing sticks. Add the tomatoes, kidney beans and stock. Bring to a gentle simmer and cook for 15–20 minutes, until the quinoa is tender. Add a dash of water if the mixture looks like drying out before it has cooked.

3. Taste and tweak the seasoning to your liking with some ground black pepper, chilli flakes and a little salt if needed.

4. Divide the chilli between two deep bowls and top with some sliced avocado and a sprinkling of chopped coriander. Serve with fat lime wedges for squeezing over.

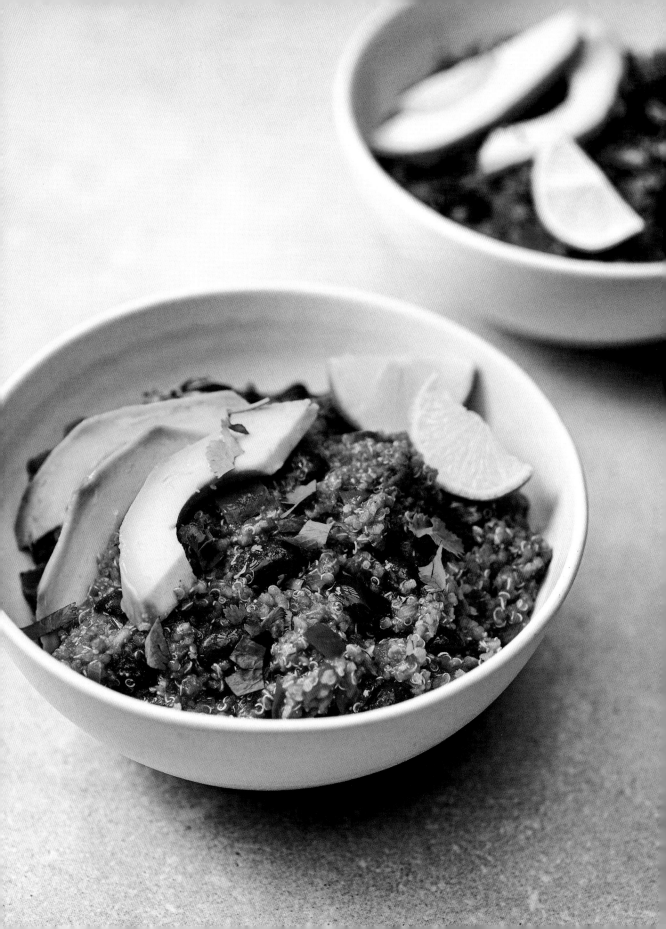

EPIC NUT ROAST WITH ONION MISO GRAVY

Perfect for a Sunday roast, or even Christmas Day, just serve this alongside some roast potatoes, carrots and greens. You can switch around the type of nuts in this recipe, as long as they add up to 200g (7oz or 1½ cups).

Serves 4

Prep & cook: 1 hour

PLANT SCORE: 11
FIBRE PER SERVING: 11g
PROTEIN PER SERVING: 15g
GLUTEN-FREE: YES, IF USING TAMARI RATHER THAN SOY SAUCE

1 tbsp extra virgin olive oil (optional)

1 celery stick, finely chopped

100g (1½ cups) chestnut mushrooms, coarsely grated or finely chopped

200g (2 cups) butternut squash, coarsely grated

50g (⅓ cup) quinoa, rinsed

150ml (⅔ cup) vegetable stock

120g (generous ½ cup) canned Puy lentils or green lentils

60g (½ cup) walnuts, roughly chopped

60g (½ cup) skinned hazelnuts, roughly chopped

80g (⅓ cup) cooked chestnuts, roughly chopped

1 garlic clove, finely chopped

2 tbsp tamari or soy sauce

1 tbsp tomato purée

1 tbsp balsamic vinegar

½ tbsp chopped fresh rosemary leaves

1 tsp fresh thyme leaves

1 tsp ground coriander

Sea salt and freshly ground black pepper

FOR THE GRAVY

1 red onion, finely sliced

1 tbsp brown rice miso

500ml (2 cups) vegetable stock

1 tbsp cornflour

Red wine vinegar, to taste

1. Preheat the oven to 180°C/Fan 160°C/350°F/Gas 4.

2. Warm the oil (if using) or a few tablespoons water in a large saucepan. Add the celery and cook gently for 5 minutes, until starting to soften.

3. Add the mushrooms and squash and continue to cook gently for another 10 minutes, until they have started to soften. Add a dash more water if they look like catching in the pan.

4. Pour in the quinoa and stock and bring to a simmer. Cook for 10–12 minutes, until the quinoa is tender and almost all the stock has been absorbed.

5. Remove from the heat and add all the remaining ingredients, stirring well to break up the lentils. Taste and tweak to your liking with a little salt and pepper, if needed.

6. Transfer the mixture to a 500g (1lb) loaf tin. Use a fork to flatten and furrow the top. Place in the oven for 30 minutes, or until slightly coloured and crisp on the top.

7. Meanwhile, make the gravy. Put the onions in a saucepan with 4 tablespoons water and cook over a gentle heat for 15 minutes, until completely soft and starting to colour. Add a dash more water if they look like catching at any point.

8. Stir in the miso, add the stock and bring to a gentle simmer.

9. In a small bowl, mix the cornflour with just enough cold water to form a paste. Stir this into the gravy and return it to a simmer until thickened. (Use more cornflour if you like a thicker gravy.) Taste and season with salt and pepper. If you think it needs a bit of sharpness, add a small dash of red wine vinegar.

10. Remove the nut roast from the oven and set aside to cool for 5 minutes. Run a knife around the sides, then turn it onto a board and serve in generous slices.

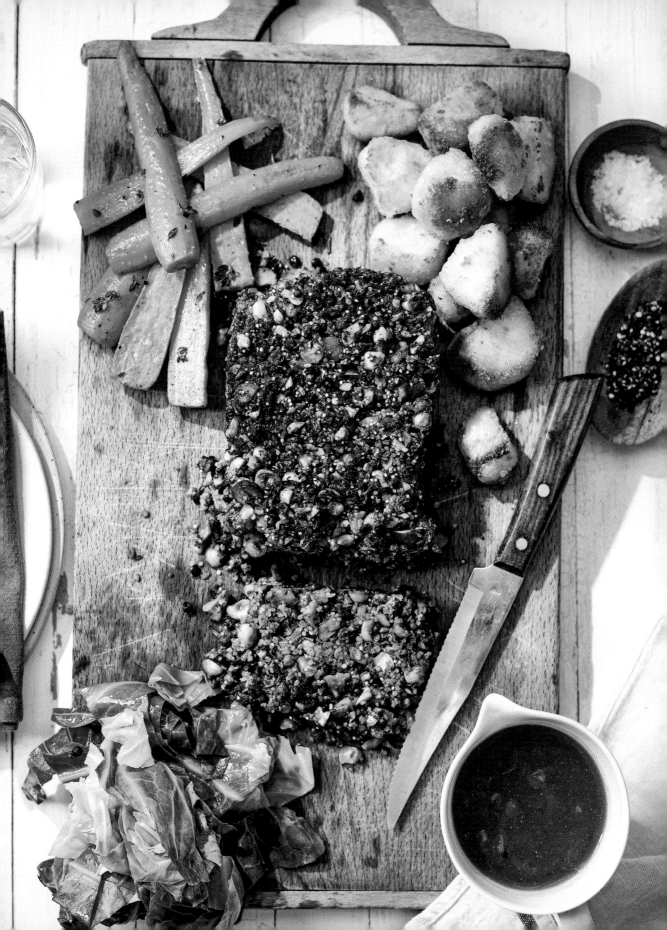

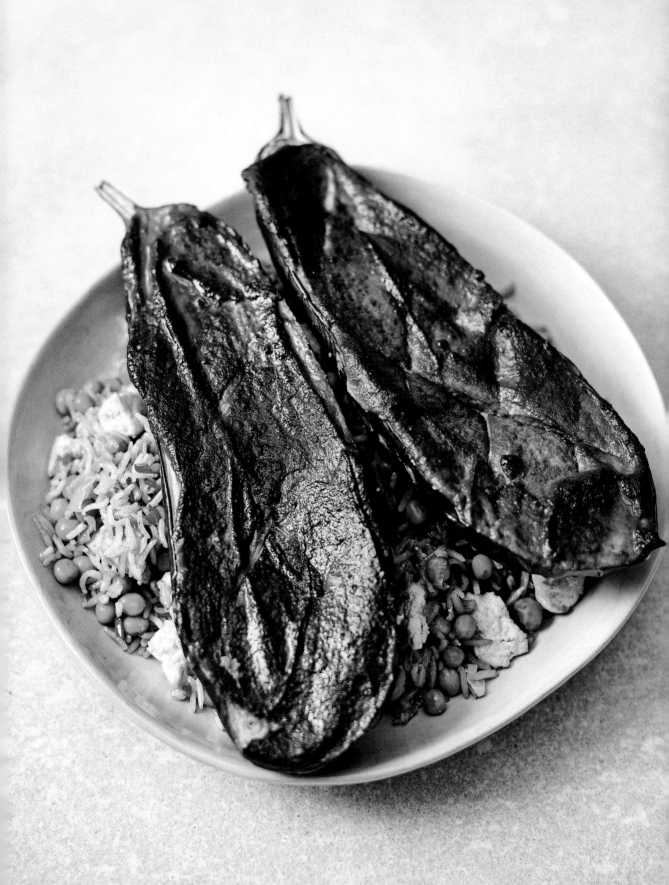

MISO AUBERGINES WITH TOFU FRIED RICE

The savoury flavours in this dish are incredible. To work well the rice needs to be cooked and cooled ahead of time. You'll need about 120g (⅔ cup) raw rice to produce 300g (1½ cups) cooked rice. Cool it under cold running water and drain completely before using. To save some time, you could just use packs of ready-cooked rice.

Serves 2
Prep & cook: 45 minutes

PLANT SCORE: 10
FIBRE PER SERVING: 11g
PROTEIN PER SERVING: 27g
GLUTEN-FREE: YES, IF USING TAMARI RATHER THAN SOY SAUCE

2 tbsp brown rice miso

2 tbsp tahini

1 tbsp rice wine vinegar

1 tbsp hot water

2 aubergines

150g (5oz) firm or extra-firm tofu, coarsely chopped

60g (½ cup) frozen peas

3 spring onions, finely sliced

2 garlic cloves, finely chopped

½ tbsp finely grated fresh root ginger

1 red chilli, deseeded and finely sliced

300g (1½ cups) cooked and cooled brown basmati rice

1 tbsp tamari or soy sauce

1 lime

1. Preheat the oven to 190ºC/Fan 170ºC/375ºF/Gas 5.

2. Put the miso, tahini, vinegar and water in a bowl and mix to make a thick paste.

3. Cut the aubergines in half lengthways and make deep criss-cross slashes in the flesh. Sit them in a roasting tray, cut side up, then divide the miso mixture between them, spreading it evenly over the surface of each one. Pour 4 tablespoons water in the bottom of the tray and cover it with foil. Transfer to the oven and bake for 25 minutes, then remove the foil and cook for a further 15–20 minutes, or until the aubergines are dark, sticky and tender.

4. When the aubergines are nearly ready, put a dry non-stick frying pan over a medium-high heat. Add the tofu and fry for 2–3 minutes, until starting to colour slightly. Add the peas, onions, garlic, ginger, chilli and 2 tablespoons water. Cook for 2 minutes before adding the rice and tamari. Cook for 2–3 minutes, stirring constantly, until the rice is piping hot and everything is cooked through. Add a dash of water if it looks like catching. Finish with a squeeze of lime juice.

5. Pile the rice into shallow bowls and sit the aubergines on top to serve.

TAHINI CAULIFLOWER WITH GREEK BULGUR WHEAT

Slicing the cauliflower gives plenty of surface area for the marinade to be absorbed and allows better contact with the roasting tray. The bulgur is best served warm, as a contrast to the piping hot cauliflower.

Serves 2
Prep & cook: 30 minutes + 30 minutes marinating

PLANT SCORE: 11
FIBRE PER SERVING: 14g
PROTEIN PER SERVING: 20g
GLUTEN-FREE: YES, IF THE BULGUR IS OMITTED; REPLACE WITH A CAN OF CHICKPEAS, DRAINED, RINSED AND COARSELY CHOPPED

1 cauliflower

100g (⅔ cup) bulgur wheat

½ tsp dried oregano

3 tomatoes, roughly chopped

½ cucumber, finely diced

½ red onion, finely diced

50g (½ cup) pitted Kalamata olives, halved

Small handful of fresh parsley, finely chopped

6 fresh mint leaves, finely chopped

1 tbsp red wine vinegar

FOR THE MARINADE

2½ tbsp tahini

Juice of 1 lemon

3 garlic cloves, finely chopped

½ tbsp smoked paprika

Sea salt and freshly ground black pepper

1. First make the marinade. Put the tahini, lemon juice, garlic and paprika in a bowl, season lightly with salt and pepper and mix well. It might look as if the lemon juice has curdled the tahini, but don't worry – it will all come together. Add a little water to thin it out if needed.

2. Trim the cauliflower and cut it in half. Cut each half into 15mm (¾ inch) slices. Add them to the marinade and turn to coat well. Set aside for at least 30 minutes.

3. Preheat the oven to 220ºC/Fan 200ºC/425ºF/Gas 7. Boil a kettleful of water.

4. Place the bulgur and oregano in a heatproof jug or bowl and pour in enough boiling water to cover by about 2cm (¾ inch). Cover with clingfilm and set aside to plump up.

5. Meanwhile, tip the cauliflower and marinade into a roasting tray and place in the oven for 15–20 minutes, turning halfway through, until golden and tender.

6. When the cauliflower is ready, mix the bulgur with the tomatoes, cucumber, onion, olives, fresh herbs and vinegar. Taste and tweak to your liking with black pepper, a little salt and some more vinegar if needed. Pile onto plates and top with the roasted cauliflower to serve.

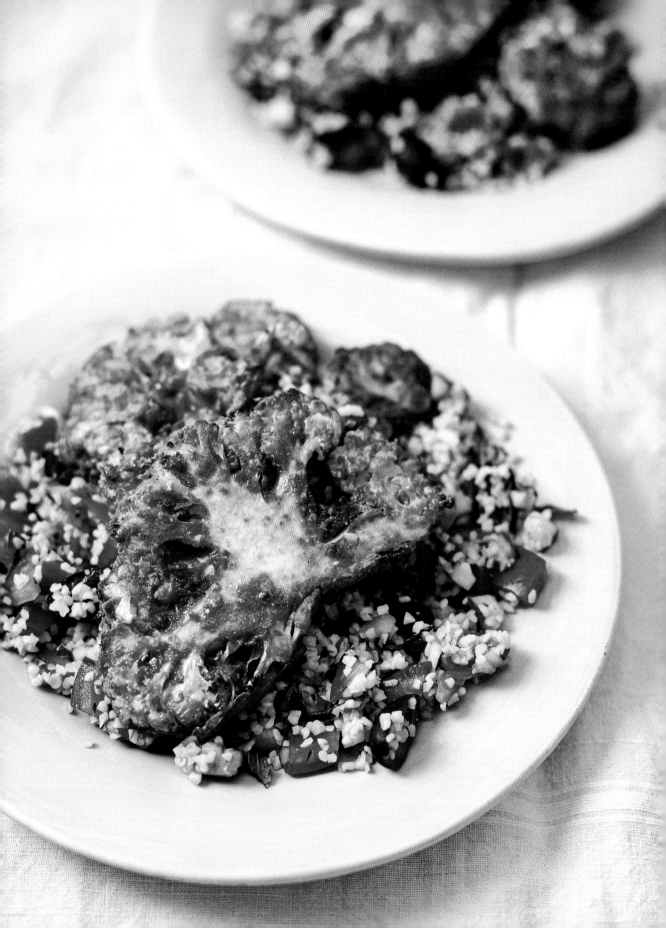

AUTUMN ROASTING TRAY TEMPEH

Who said that plants don't contain protein! Make sure to cover the squash for the first half of cooking. Once the cover is off, the veg then can roast to perfection alongside the marinaded tempeh.

Serves 2
Prep & cook: 45 minutes

PLANT SCORE: 9
FIBRE PER SERVING: 25g
PROTEIN PER SERVING: 46g
GLUTEN-FREE: YES, IF USING TAMARI RATHER THAN SOY SAUCE

2 garlic cloves, roughly chopped

2 tbsp tamari or soy sauce

1 tbsp balsamic vinegar

½ tsp smoked paprika

200g (¾ cup) tempeh, cut into 2cm (¾ inch) cubes

1 butternut squash, peeled, deseeded and cut into 2.5cm (1 inch) chunks

3 Portobello mushrooms, thickly sliced

1 red onion, sliced

1 tbsp extra virgin olive oil (optional)

½ tbsp chopped fresh rosemary

30g (¼ cup) roughly chopped walnuts

200ml (¾ cup) vegetable stock

120g (2½ cups) black kale, stalks removed and roughly sliced

1 x 400g (14oz) can Puy lentils, drained and rinsed

Sea salt and freshly ground black pepper

1. Put the garlic, tamari, vinegar and paprika in a shallow bowl and mix well. Add the tempeh and turn to coat. Set aside to marinate.

2. Preheat the oven to 200ºC/Fan 180ºC/400ºF/Gas 6. Throw the squash, mushrooms and onion into a large roasting tray with the oil (if using) and 2 tablespoons water. Season lightly with salt and pepper, mix well and cover the tray with foil. Place in the oven for 15 minutes.

3. Remove the foil and scatter the tempeh and its marinade over the squash. Return to the oven for another 15–20 minutes, until the squash is tender and the tempeh is nicely coloured and starting to crisp around the edges. Add the rosemary and walnuts for the final 5 minutes of cooking time.

4. Meanwhile, place the stock and kale in a saucepan, bring to a simmer and cook for 2–3 minutes, until the kale has started to wilt. Add the lentils and cook gently for 5 minutes, until they have warmed through and the kale is completely soft.

5. To serve, pile the lentil mixture onto plates and top with the roasted vegetables.

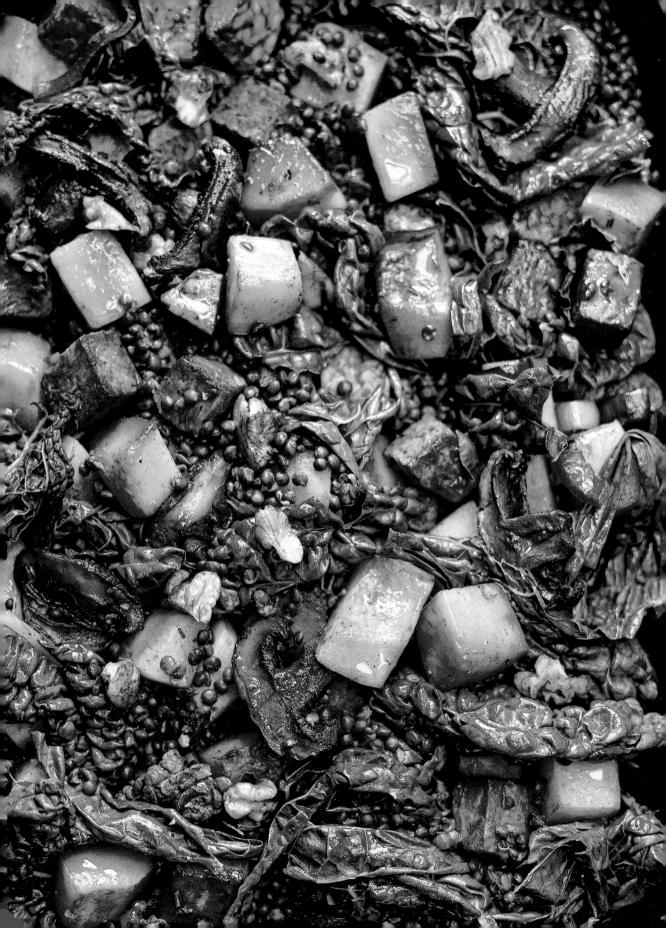

SWEET TREATS

The big fruit bowl with sweet tahini dip **176**

Barbecued fruits **178**

Dreamy hot chocolate **180**

Carrot cake bites **180**

Apple and apricot crumble **182**

Chocolate beanie brownies **184**

Frozen treats **186**

Glorious summer pudding **190**

Cherry cacao bars **192**

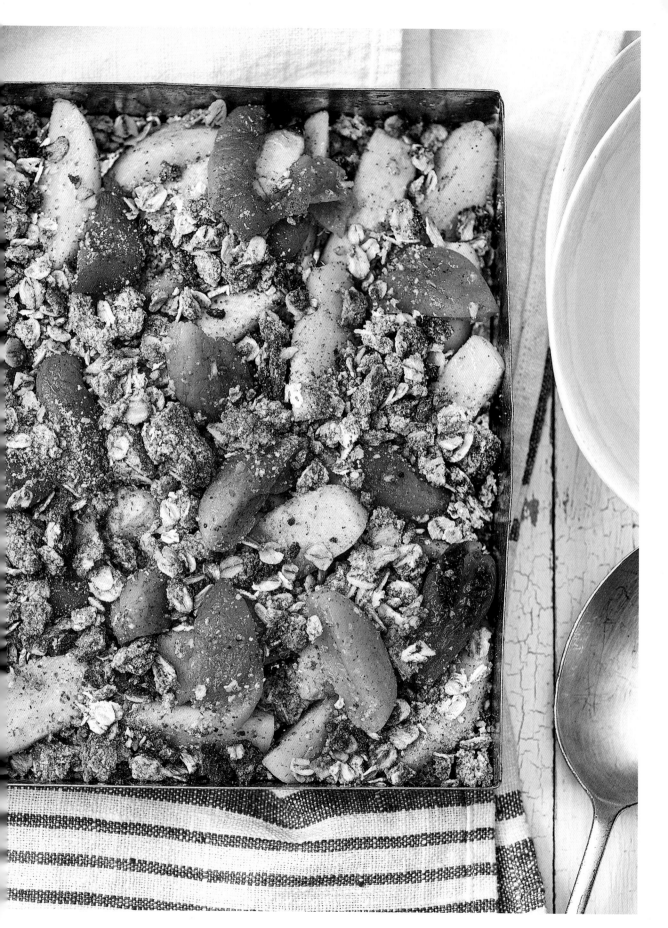

THE BIG FRUIT BOWL WITH SWEET TAHINI DIP

My favourite sweet treat is always some fresh fruit. Sometimes it's nice to make it an occasion by serving up a big bowl. The sweet tahini dip gives the healthiest of desserts a sweet and satisfying lift.

Serves 2
Prep time: 5 minutes

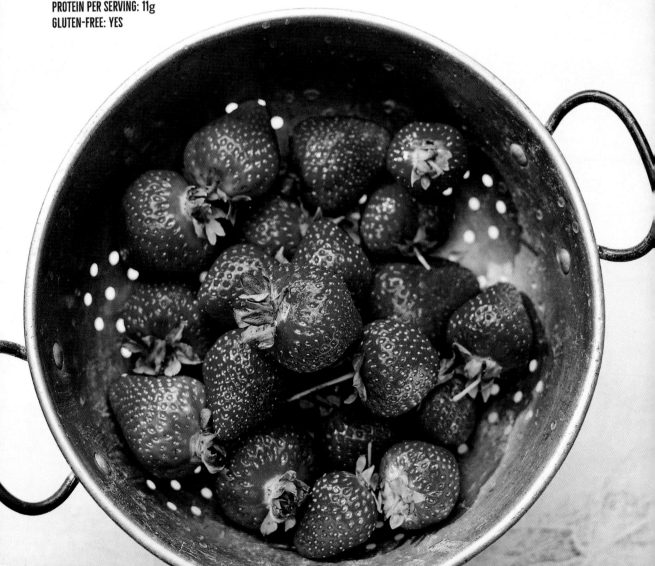

PLANT SCORE: 2+
FIBRE PER SERVING: 2.7g
PROTEIN PER SERVING: 11g
GLUTEN-FREE: YES

3 tbsp tahini

250ml (1 cup) natural soy or other plant-based yogurt

2 tbsp maple syrup

Pinch of ground cinnamon

1. Stir the ingredients together in a small bowl. Serve with a plate of any chopped fruits: apples, pears, bananas, grapes, strawberries or whatever takes you fancy.

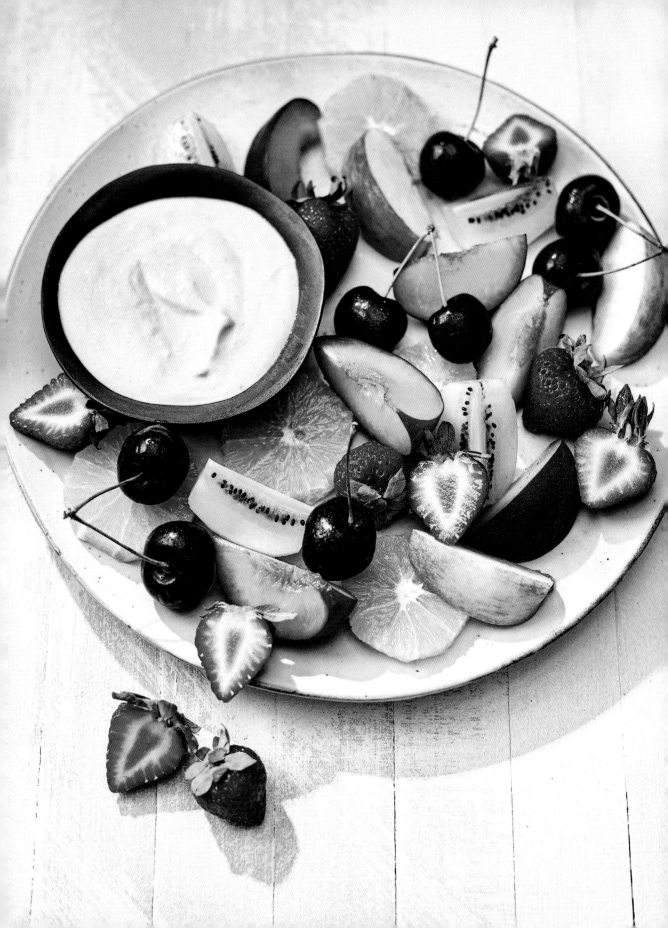

BARBECUED FRUITS

These caramelised fruits are a perfect finish to a summer barbecue. Serve on their own, or with a scoop of homemade ice cream (see page 186).

Each recipe makes 2 servings

NECTARINES & ALMONDS

Prep & cook: 12-15 minutes

PLANT SCORE: 2
FIBRE PER SERVING: 5.6g
PROTEIN PER SERVING: 5.2g
GLUTEN-FREE: YES

3 nectarines, halved and stoned

Zest and juice of 1 small orange

25g (⅓ cup) flaked and toasted almonds

1. Halve the nectarines and remove the stones. Place the fruit cut side down on a medium-hot barbecue or griddle for 4–5 minutes, until nicely marked. Turn them over and cook for 4 more minutes, until the flesh is soft and the skin is starting to pull away from it. (Don't forget to eat the skin – the best part!)

2. Divide the fruit between 2 bowls and drizzle each with 2 spoonfuls of the orange juice. Sprinkle with the almonds and orange zest before serving.

WATERMELON & MINT

Prep & cook: 10 minutes

PLANT SCORE: 2
FIBRE PER SERVING: 1.1g
PROTEIN PER SERVING: 1.3g
GLUTEN-FREE: YES

6 large fresh mint leaves

Zest and juice of 1 lime

½ small watermelon

1. Finely chop the mint leaves with the lime zest and keep to one side.

2. Cut the watermelon into 2cm (¾ inch) slices. Remove the seeds and place the slices on a hot barbecue or griddle and cook for about 1 minute on each side, until you see charred lines on the fruit.

3. Cut the slices into wedges, place in bowls and sprinkle with the mint and lime mixture. Finish with a little lime juice and eat immediately.

STRAWBERRIES & BALSAMIC

Prep & cook: 10 minutes

PLANT SCORE: 1
FIBRE PER SERVING: 4.7g
PROTEIN PER SERVING: 0.8g
GLUTEN-FREE: YES

250g (scant 3 cups) strawberries

2 tbsp balsamic vinegar

1. Hull the strawberries, cut any very large ones in half, and keep the rest whole. Put them in a bowl with the vinegar, mix well and set aside for 5 minutes.

2. When your barbecue or griddle is medium-hot, add the strawberries, leaving the vinegar in the bowl. Griddle for 1–2 minutes, turning once or twice, until lightly marked and starting to soften.

3. Divide the fruit between 2 bowls and spoon any remaining vinegar over the top. Eat immediately.

MANGO & COCONUT

Prep & cook: 10 minutes

PLANT SCORE: 2
FIBRE 8.2g
PROTEIN 2.2g
GLUTEN-FREE: YES

2 large mangoes, peeled, stoned and thickly sliced

1 lime

1½ tbsp toasted coconut flakes

1. Place the mango slices on a hot barbecue rack or griddle and cook for 1–2 minutes on each side, until caramelised and nicely marked. Serve hot with a squeeze of lime juice and some coconut flakes to garnish.

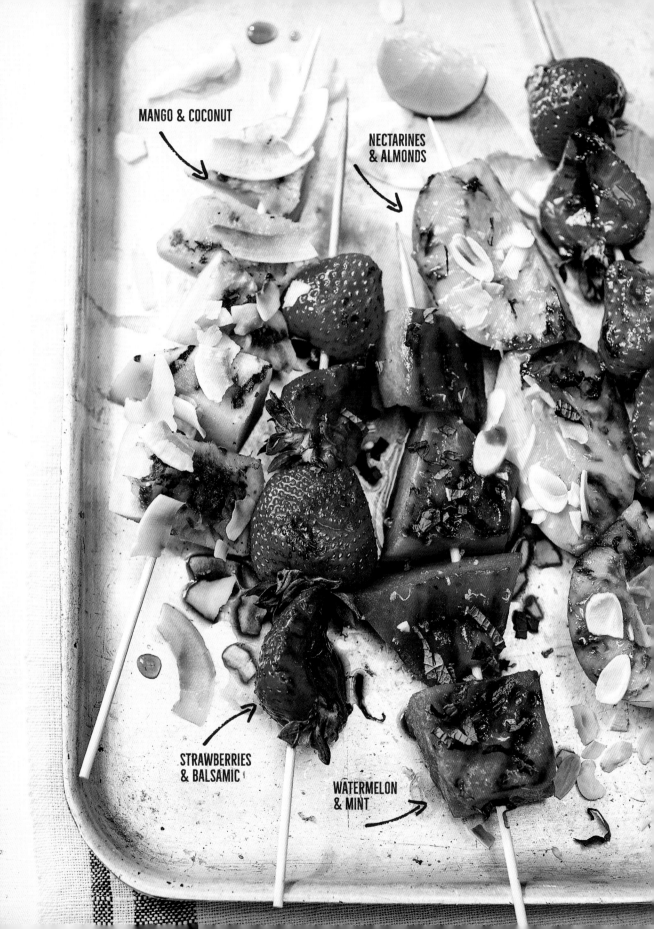

MANGO & COCONUT

NECTARINES & ALMONDS

STRAWBERRIES & BALSAMIC

WATERMELON & MINT

DREAMY HOT CHOCOLATE

This recipe uses the natural sweetness of dates to deliver a proper cup of chocolate indulgence.

Serves 2
Prep & cook: 10 minutes

PLANT SCORE: 2
FIBRE PER SERVING: 8.5g
PROTEIN PER SERVING: 5.4g
GLUTEN-FREE: YES

400ml (1¾ cups) almond milk, or any plant-based milk

4 pitted Medjool dates

2 tbsp raw cacao powder, plus more to sprinkle

¼ tsp ground cinnamon, plus more to taste

½ tsp vanilla extract

1. Place the milk in a large saucepan with the dates and cacao. Bring to a simmer and leave over the heat for 3 minutes.

2. Tip the mixture into a blender and add the cinnamon and vanilla. Blitz until completely smooth, then divide between 2 mugs. Sprinkle with some extra cacao to finish.

CARROT CAKE BITES

These healthy snacks take just ten minutes to make. You can experiment by changing the nuts and adding some dark chocolate, seeds or chopped dried fruit in place of the carrot.

Makes 12
Prep: 10 minutes

PLANT SCORE: 4
FIBRE PER SERVING: 3.1g
PROTEIN PER SERVING: 3.4g
GLUTEN-FREE: YES, IF USING GLUTEN-FREE OATS

125g (1 cup) walnut halves

120g (1½ cups) porridge oats

10 pitted Medjool dates

1 carrot, grated

1 tbsp maple syrup (optional)

1 tsp ground cinnamon

¼ tsp ground nutmeg

1. Put the walnuts into a food processor or blender and pulse them a few times until coarsely chopped. Add all the remaining ingredients and whizz together until you have a thick, sticky dough.

2. Scrape the dough onto a sheet of baking parchment. Wet your hands and roll the dough into a sausage shape. If it feels too sticky to shape, return it to the processor and add more oats until it is easier to handle. Cut the sausage into 12 equal pieces, then roll each one into a ball. Store them in a covered container in the fridge for up to a week.

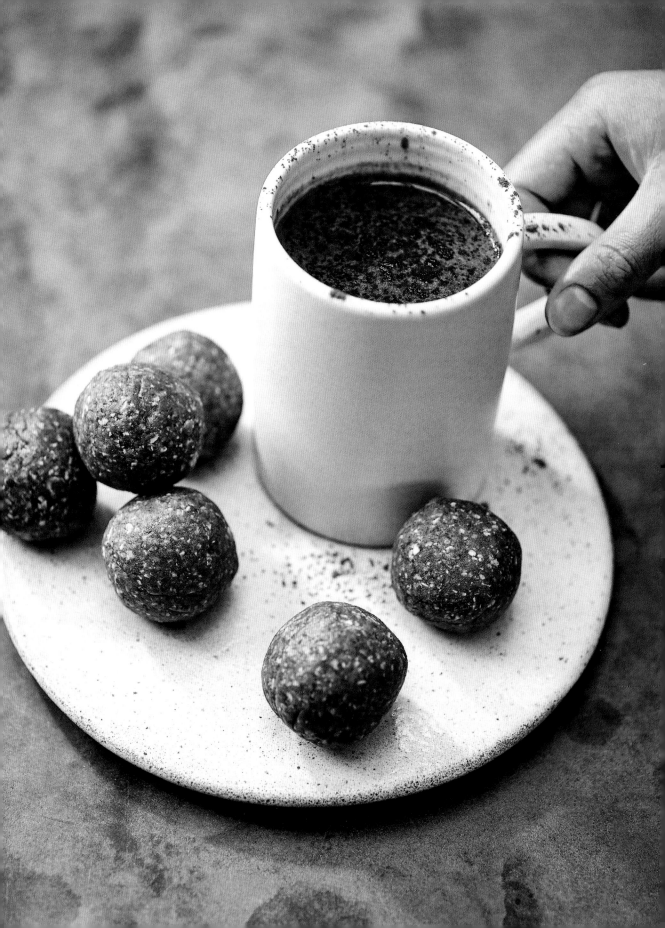

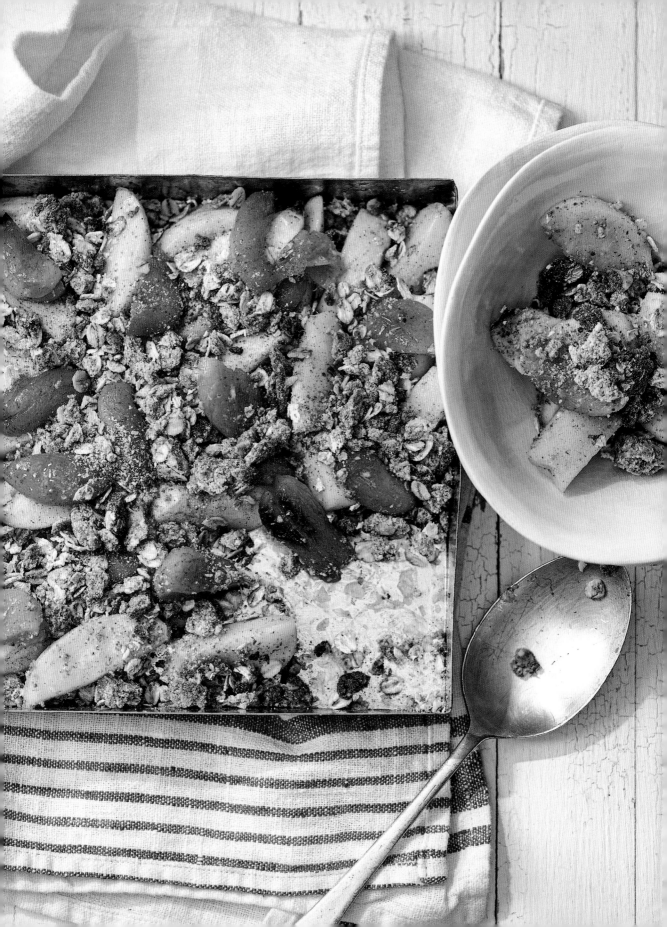

APPLE & APRICOT CRUMBLE

The perfect plant-based comfort food. You can change the fruit in your crumble depending on the time of year. Making sure that at least half the total quantity is apple tends to work well. Try it served with a cool scoop of Banana pecan ice cream (page 186).

Serves 4
Prep & cook: 50 minutes

PLANT SCORE: 5
FIBRE PER SERVING: 2.7g
PROTEIN PER SERVING: 11g
GLUTEN-FREE: YES, IF USING GLUTEN-FREE
FLOUR AND OATS

80g (generous ½ cup) dried apricots, roughly chopped

4 tbsp boiling water

500g (about 3) eating apples, peeled, cored and cut into 2cm (¾ inch) pieces

¼ tsp ground cinnamon

FOR THE TOPPING

60g (⅓ cup + 1 tbsp) wholemeal flour (or gluten-free flour)

30g (¼ cup) ground almonds

60g (⅓ cup) rolled oats

1 tbsp extra virgin olive oil (optional)

2 tbsp maple syrup, plus 1 extra tbsp if not using the oil

1. Preheat the oven to 180°C/Fan 160°C/350°F/Gas 4.

2. Place the apricots in a heatproof bowl and add the boiling water. Set aside to soak for 10 minutes.

3. Tip the apricots and their liquid into a baking tray (about 18 x 18cm) with the apples and cinnamon. Mix well.

4. To make the topping, combine all the ingredients in a large bowl, adding an extra tablespoon maple syrup if not using the oil. Use your hands to rub the mixture into coarse crumbs. Sprinkle evenly over the fruit, then wet your hands and flick the water on them over the crumble – this prevents it from browning too fast before the fruit has cooked.

5. Transfer the tray to the oven and bake for 30 minutes, or until golden on top and bubbling beneath.

6. Serve with a scoop of Banana pecan ice cream (see page 186), or a dollop of plant-based yogurt.

CHOCOLATE BEANIE BROWNIES

Black beans are the secret ingredient that make these brownies nutritious, satisfying and extra fudgy. Your friends will never believe that you've just added to their daily intake of legumes!

Makes 8
Prep & cook: 40 minutes

PLANT SCORE: 7
FIBRE PER SERVING: 8.1g
PROTEIN PER SERVING: 6.8g
GLUTEN-FREE: YES, IF USING GLUTEN-FREE FLOUR

3 Medjool dates, roughly chopped

5 tbsp boiling water

75g (½ cup) plain wholemeal flour

1 tsp baking powder

30g (3 tbsp) cacao nibs, or chopped dairy-free dark chocolate

50g (⅓ cup) toasted and chopped hazelnuts

1x 400g (14oz) can black beans, drained and rinsed

2 bananas (about 150g/5oz in total), peeled and sliced

4 tbsp raw cacao powder

1. Place the dates in a bowl and add the boiling water. Set aside for 10 minutes to soften.

2. Meanwhile, preheat the oven to 180°C/Fan 160°C/350°F/Gas 4. Line a square baking tin (18 x 18cm) with baking parchment.

3. Sift the flour and baking powder into a large bowl, returning the husks after sifting. Stir in the cacao nibs and hazelnuts.

4. Tip the dates and their liquid into a food processor or blender along with the beans, bananas and cacao powder. Blitz together until smooth, scraping down the sides of the bowl or jug a couple of times to catch every last bit.

5. Add the purée to the flour and gently fold together, until well combined with no obvious lumps. Don't overmix or beat it or you'll end up with a flat, cakey brownie.

6. Pour the batter into the prepared tin and level it out with a spatula. Bake for 25 minutes, or until the tip of a knife inserted in the middle comes out clean.

7. Set aside to cool completely in the tin, then turn out and cut into 8 squares. If not eating straight away, store in an airtight container in the fridge for up to 3 days.

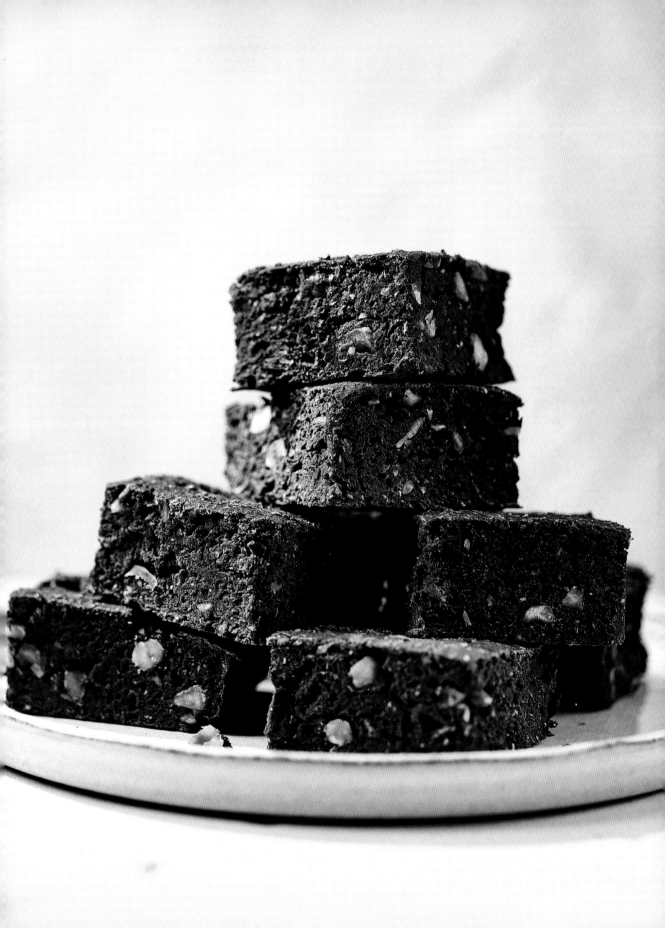

FROZEN TREATS

Everyone loves an ice-cold treat on a hot day. Here are four simple ideas with fruit at their heart.

BANANA PECAN ICE CREAM

You'll be amazed at how creamy and sweet this ice cream is. Stockpile your overripe bananas ahead of time: simply peel and chop them into 2cm (¾ inch) slices, place in a plastic container and keep in the freezer until the sun comes out.

Serves 2
Prep: 10 minutes + overnight freezing

PLANT SCORE: 2
FIBRE PER SERVING: 2.6g
PROTEIN PER SERVING: 3g
GLUTEN-FREE: YES

30g (¼ cup) pecan nuts, roughly chopped

2 large ripe bananas, peeled and sliced into 2cm (¾ inch) pieces, frozen overnight

1 tbsp maple syrup (optional)

1. Put the pecans in a dry pan over a medium heat and toast them, stirring frequently, until golden brown; take care not to burn them. Transfer them to a plate and set aside to cool.

2. Put the frozen banana slices into a food processor or blender with the maple syrup (if using) and blitz until smooth. It doesn't look like it's working at first, but stay with it and the bananas will change from frozen chunks into a creamy mass. You might need to stop occasionally and scrape down the sides of the bowl or jug.

3. When the mixture looks nice and creamy, transfer it to a small plastic container and fold the toasted pecans through it. Freeze for 10 minutes before serving. This sweet treat will keep in your freezer for weeks, but remember to take it out 10 minutes before serving so that it softens slightly and is easier to scoop.

RASPBERRY RIPPLE ICE CREAM

PLANT SCORE: 2
FIBRE PER SERVING: 4.8g
PROTEIN PER SERVING: 2g
GLUTEN-FREE: YES

Use the banana pecan recipe but leave out the pecan nuts. Instead, place 100g (⅔ cup) raspberries in a small saucepan with 1 tablespoon water and heat gently for a few minutes until the fruit breaks down. Use the back of a spoon to press them into a rough sauce. Set aside to cool completely, then pour the raspberries into the container of ice cream and use a spoon to ripple them through it at step 3. Refreeze for 10 minutes before serving.

CHOCOLATE CHIP ICE CREAM

PLANT SCORE: 2
FIBRE PER SERVING: 4.6g
PROTEIN PER SERVING: 3.6g
GLUTEN-FREE: YES

For chocolate chip, use the same recipe without the pecans. Add 1 tablespoon raw cacao powder to the bananas when you blend them. Fold ½ tablespoon cacao nibs or 1 tablespoon chopped dairy-free chocolate through the ice cream at step 3, once it's in the plastic container and ready to freeze.

MANGO SORBET

Depending how ripe your mangoes are, you might not need to sweeten this sorbet at all. Try to use fruits that are a little overripe as they tend to be completely sweet and soft.

Makes 4 servings
Prep: 15 minutes plus overnight freeze

PLANT SCORE: 1
FIBRE PER SERVING: 2.9g
PROTEIN PER SERVING: 0.8g
GLUTEN-FREE: YES

2 large ripe mangoes, peeled, stoned and diced

125ml (½ cup) plant milk (coconut works really well with the mango)

Juice of 1 lime

Maple syrup (optional)

1. Lay the diced mango on a baking tray in a single layer and put in the freezer overnight.

2. Put the frozen mango into a food processor or blender, add the milk and half the lime juice and blitz until smooth. It doesn't look like it is working at first, but stay with it. You might need to stop occasionally and scrape down the sides of the bowl or jug.

3. Taste the sorbet and add more lime juice and some maple syrup if you think they're needed. Transfer to a plastic container and place in the freezer for 10 minutes before serving. If not eating straight away, this sorbet will keep for weeks in the freezer, but take it out 10 minutes before scooping.

STRAWBERRY MINI MILKS

The classic childhood ice lolly!

Fills 4 x 100ml (½ cup) ice lolly moulds
Prep: 10 minutes plus overnight freeze

PLANT SCORE: 1
FIBRE PER SERVING: 2.4g
PROTEIN PER SERVING: 0.9g
GLUTEN-FREE: YES

300g (2 cups) strawberries

200ml (¾ cup) almond milk

1 tbsp maple syrup (optional)

1. Hull the strawberries, then place them in a food processor or blender. Add the other ingredients and blitz until smooth. If you prefer an even smoother mixture, push it through a sieve.

2. Divide the mixture between 4 moulds, insert the sticks and freeze.

APPLE & BLACKBERRY ICE LOLLIES

A late summer treat, these lollies would ideally be made with freshly pressed apple juice and blackberries straight from the wild. Failing that, shop-bought ingredients are pretty good too. The recipe also works well with raspberries or strawberries.

Fills 4 x 100ml (½ cup) ice lolly moulds
Prep: 10 minutes plus overnight freeze

PLANT SCORE: 1
FIBRE PER SERVING: 5.3g
PROTEIN PER SERVING: 0.8g
GLUTEN-FREE: YES

200ml (¾ cup) cloudy apple juice

300g (2¼ cups) fresh blackberries

1. Put the juice and fruit into a food processor or blender and blitz until smooth. For an even smoother mixture, push it through a sieve.

2. Divide the mixture between 4 moulds, insert the sticks and freeze.

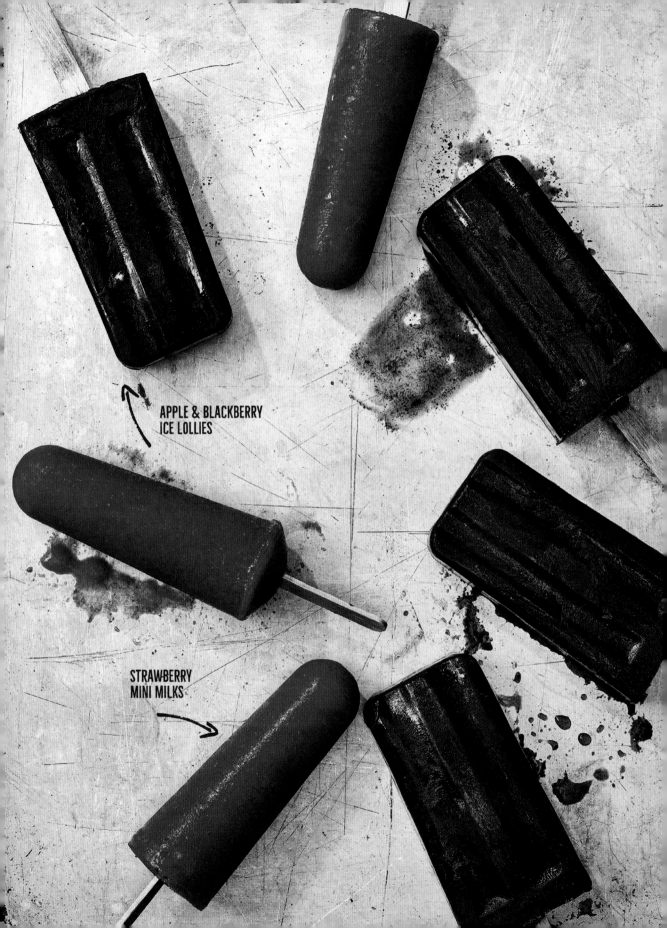

APPLE & BLACKBERRY
ICE LOLLIES

STRAWBERRY
MINI MILKS

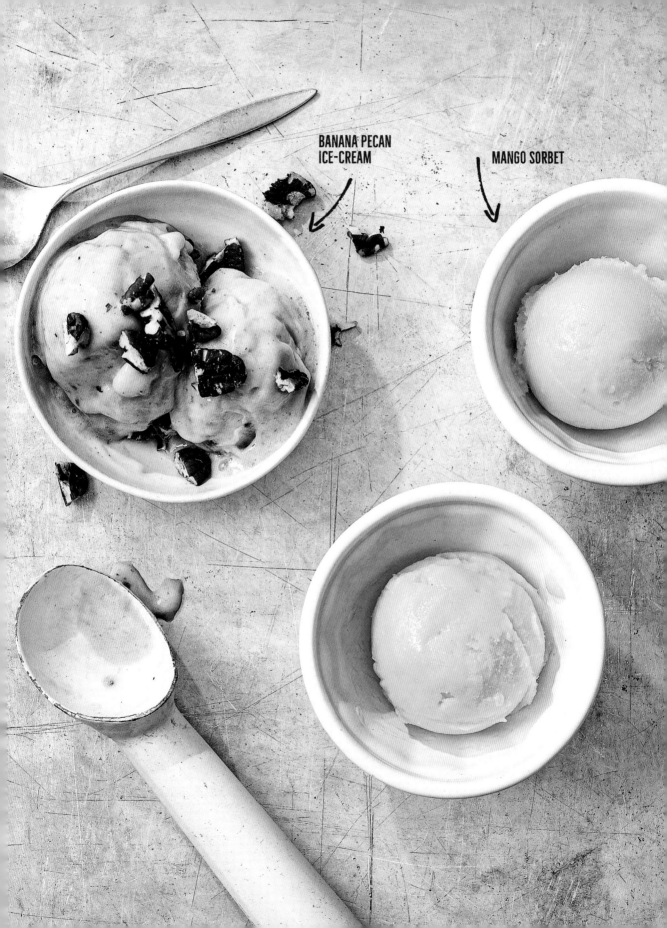

BANANA PECAN
ICE-CREAM

MANGO SORBET

GLORIOUS SUMMER PUDDING

Here's a classic pud, and simplicity itself to make. Fresh fruit is ideal, but frozen berry mixtures are easily available. Avoid using bread that is full of seeds and nuts as it can spoil the deliciously soggy texture.

Serves 2–3 (fills a 500ml/2 cup pudding bowl)
Prep: 20 minutes + overnight freezing

PLANT SCORE: 5
FIBRE PER SERVING: 9.3g
PROTEIN PER SERVING: 13g
GLUTEN-FREE: NO

400g (2⅓ cups) mixed summer berries, defrosted if frozen

2 tbsp maple syrup

5 slices of wholegrain bread, crusts removed

FOR THE CASHEW CREAM

100g (¾ cup) raw unsalted cashew nuts

1 tsp maple syrup

1. Place the fruit in a small saucepan with the maple syrup and warm gently for a couple of minutes, until it begins to soften a little. Set aside.

2. Line a 500ml (2 cup) bowl or pudding basin with clingfilm, making sure it overhangs the side.

3. Cut one slice of bread into a circle and press it into the bottom of the bowl. Use 3 slices to line the sides of the bowl, overlapping and pressing them down to make sure there aren't any gaps.

4. Tip the fruit and all its liquid into the bowl. Place the final slice of bread on top, trimming it to fit. Lift the overhanging clingfilm and use it to cover the surface of the pudding. Sit a saucer on top.

5. Place the bowl in a tray (to catch any juices) and sit a heavy weight (such as a can of beans) on the saucer to press everything down. Place in the fridge overnight.

6. Put the cashew nuts in a bowl, cover with plenty of cold water and leave them in the fridge overnight too.

7. The next day, drain the cashews, then place in a blender with the maple syrup and 100ml (½ cup) fresh cold water. Blend until creamy. Taste, and if the cream is still gritty, add a splash of water and blend some more. Transfer to a covered container and store in the fridge until needed. (If you omit the maple syrup from the cashew cream, it can be used in soups and other dishes to add a savoury smoothness.)

8. To serve the pudding, remove the saucer and open the clingfilm. Place a shallow dish on top and invert both bowl and dish so that the pudding turns out in one piece. Serve generous slices with a pouring of the cashew cream.

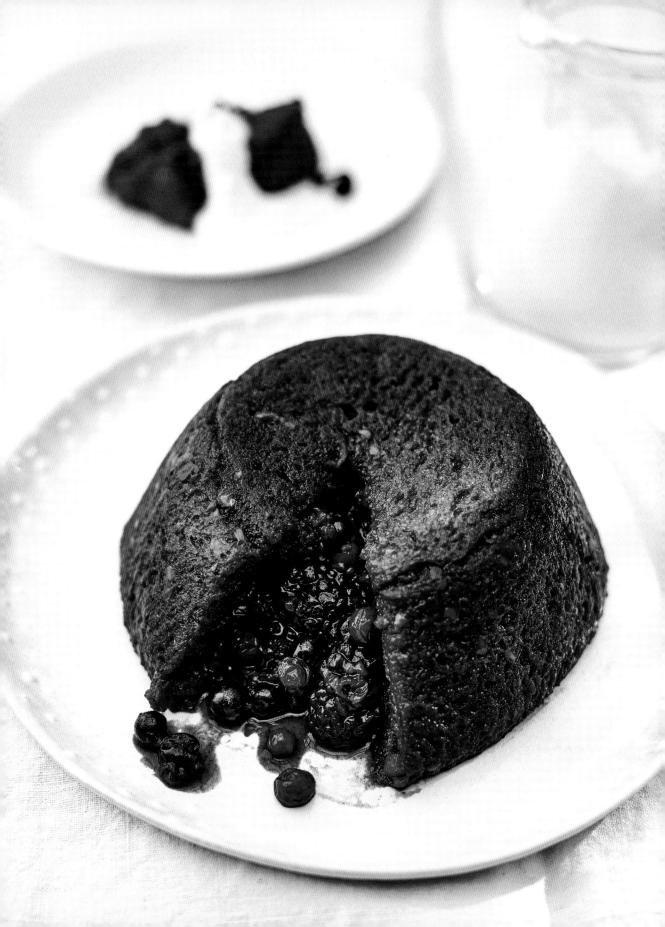

CHERRY CACAO BARS

Perfect for breakfast, with a cup of tea for elevenses, or as a sweet treat after a meal, these bars are great at any time. You can adjust the nuts, seeds and fruits to your liking, as long as you use the same proportions.

Makes 8
Prep & cook: 30 minutes + 1 hour soaking

PLANT SCORE: 8
FIBRE PER SERVING: 6.1g
PROTEIN PER SERVING: 8.5g
GLUTEN-FREE: YES, IF USING GLUTEN-FREE OATS

200g (1⅓ cups) pitted dates

½ tsp bicarbonate of soda

3 tbsp peanut or almond butter

50g (generous ½ cup) rolled oats

100g (1 cup) flaked and toasted almonds, roughly chopped

3 tbsp cacao nibs, or coarsely chopped dark chocolate

30g (¼ cup) pumpkin seeds, roughly chopped

30g (¼ cup) sunflower seeds

40g (⅓ cup) dried sour cherries

Pinch of ground cinnamon

1. Put the dates and bicarbonate of soda in a heatproof bowl and cover with boiling water. Set aside to soak for 1 hour.

2. Just before starting step 3, preheat the oven to 160°C/Fan 140°C/325°F/Gas 3. Line a small baking tray (about 18 x 18cm/7 x 7 inches) with baking parchment.

3. Drain the dates and place them in a food processor or blender with the peanut butter. Blend until you have a smooth paste.

4. Scrape the paste into a bowl and add all the remaining ingredients. Mix thoroughly with a wooden spoon.

5. Pour the mixture into the prepared tray and cover with a sheet of baking parchment. Use the back of a spoon to level and compress the mixture as much as possible. Transfer to the oven, with the parchment still on top, and bake for 20 minutes. Set aside to cool in the tin before transferring to the fridge to set.

6. When firm, run a knife around the tray, turn out the cake and cut into 8 equal pieces. This is easier if you dip your knife into boiling water between cuts – it stops the cake sticking to the knife. These bars will keep for a week in an airtight container.

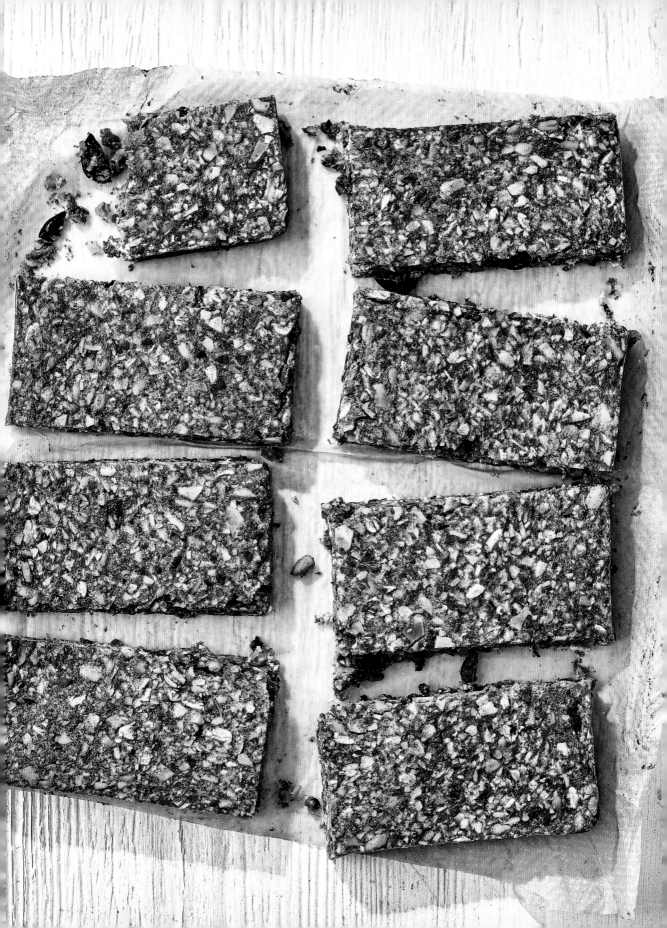

PART FOUR

THE 28-DAY REVOLUTION

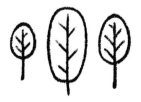

PREPARING FOR THE REVOLUTION

I hope that you've enjoyed discovering just how satisfying and flavourful healthy plant-based meals can be. If our Recipes for the Revolution have helped you to increase the number of completely plant-based meals in your average week then I'm sure you'll have already noticed some benefits. The 28-Day Revolution will push you even further, challenging you to experience how well you can feel eating a completely plant-based diet.

You've read the science. Making the switch to a plant-based diet can transform your gut microbiome, improve your digestion, promote healthy weight loss, control type 2 diabetes, fight heart disease, and even improve your mood. You now understand why so many doctors and health professionals recommend a whole-food, plant-based diet as the optimal choice for human health and longevity. It's time to try it for yourself. Twenty-eight days eating nothing but plants!

It's going to be a busy four weeks. Before you get stuck into the shopping lists and meal plans, it can be helpful to spend some time preparing for your personal 28-day revolution.

PERSONAL GOALS

Setting well-defined personal goals can be the key to success in any positive lifestyle change. The simplest way to find your personal goals is to quickly write down as many answers as you can think of to this simple question: 'Why am I joining the 28-Day Revolution?' Do it right now, I'll wait!

These goals will be highly personal and unique to you. Here are some examples of what they might look like:

I want to gain a better understanding of cooking healthy plant-based meals.

I want to eat better and encourage my children and husband to enjoy healthy food.

I want to eat more wholefoods and banish my junk food addiction.

I already enjoy plant-based meals, so now I want to go all-out to improve my general well-being.

My goals are to improve my energy levels and my relationship with food.

I love cooking and want to experiment with new ingredients.

I'd like to be healthier and reduce the environmental impact of my food choices.

I want to make a positive change and feel happier about my food and my life.

HEALTH GOALS

A whole-food, plant-based diet ticks all the right boxes for a healthier gut, heart, body and mind. If you've been diagnosed with a condition such as irritable bowel syndrome, type 2 diabetes, high blood pressure or high cholesterol, your health goals might include improved symptoms or the ability to reduce your medication. If you have any ongoing medical condition, especially type 2 diabetes or high blood pressure, please ask your healthcare team to support you as you make these healthy changes. You'll find an important letter for your GP or practice nurse on page 199. Read it for yourself and share a copy with them.

Setting goals for the next 28 days is not mandatory. The real revolution may well be the changes you experience in your mindset and your approach to meal times as you successfully move to a style of eating designed to maximise your chances of a longer and healthier life.

CALORIE COUNTING NOT REQUIRED

The 28-Day Revolution does not involve calorie counting. The science shows that it's not required. I simply want you to enjoy a variety of plant-based meals and snacks each day while eating to your natural appetite. The plan is not rigid, so you can eat more food, or less, depending on your appetite. The meal plans have been reviewed and approved by a registered dietitian and they are nutritionally complete. If you eat the meal plans exactly as they appear, you'll be eating an average of 1,750 calories, 70g of protein and 55g of fibre each day. Your average daily iron intake (15mg) and calcium intake (780mg) will also comfortably exceed the recommended daily intakes for healthy adults. The meal plan includes tips on increasing your intake of food if required. If you have specific medical or dietetic requirements, you can find detailed nutritional analysis of all the recipes and meal plans at alandesmond.com/revolution

A FEW WORDS ABOUT WEIGHT LOSS

If you are aiming for healthy weight loss, it's important to bear in mind that more is not always better. Small reductions over time are far more likely to lead to long-term success. This is not a crash diet, it's the beginning of a lifelong journey. How much your weight will change during the 28-Day Revolution depends on your starting point. To figure this out, you'll need to know your body mass index (BMI).

Your BMI is a useful measure of how close you are to a healthy weight for your height. It's not perfect, but it's easy to calculate and a good overall indicator. A quick web search for 'BMI calculator' will throw up lots of on-line tools to help you calculate yours. You'll just need to know your height and weight.

WHAT YOUR BMI NUMBER MEANS

18.5–24.9:	HEALTHY WEIGHT
25–29.9:	OVERWEIGHT
30 OR HIGHER:	OBESE

With a starting BMI in the healthy range, you might expect to lose between zero and 5% of your body weight. In fact, at this weight, one of your goals might be to hit the gym and pile on some extra muscle weight. If this is the case, the 28-Day Revolution has got you covered. The meal plans allow you to eat as much food as you need and provide more than enough healthy plant-based protein to fuel your gains.

If your starting BMI is in the overweight or obese ranges, then planning to lose 2–8% of your starting weight is reasonable. For example, a person starting with a height of 170cm (5ft 7 in) and a weight of 112kg (245lb) has a BMI of 38.7. They are in the obese range and should expect to lose 2–9kg (4–20lb) over four weeks. Remember, smaller changes are more likely to lead to long-term success.

TRACKING YOUR CHOLESTEROL LEVEL

Although your cholesterol level is just one measure of health, it's a number that is often focused on by doctors and researchers. An elevated level of non-HDL ('bad' cholesterol) puts you at increased risk of heart disease and stroke. Even people with non-HDL in the upper range of normal can benefit from lowering their number. If you already have high cholesterol, you're reading the right book! With a starting non HDL level greater than 4.0 mmol/L, you're likely to see a reduction of 15–25%. The most impressive drops I've seen in just four weeks have been 35–40%. Your doctor should be impressed.

TIME, SPACE AND SUPPORT!

It's going to be a busy four weeks as you chop, prep and cook your way to better health! To make this revolution a success, you'll need three things:

TIME. Our meal plans are designed to allow you to cook just four times per week. You may initially find that you are spending more time in the kitchen than usual, but you'll soon become more efficient and settle into the new routine. It's best not to take on the 28-Day Revolution the same month that you are moving to a new house, getting married or starting a business! Chose a four-week period when you know you'll have time. If you have a supportive friend or family member to help with some of the cooking, all the better.

SPACE. The shopping lists include all the ingredients you'll need to cook your breakfast, lunch and dinner for 28 days, plus some sweet treats and fresh fruit. You'll need plenty of storage space in your cupboards and fridge. It's a good idea to have extra airtight containers on hand to freeze any leftovers for later.

SUPPORT. Share your plans with friends and family. If you feel comfortable doing so, also share your goals with the people who value your health and happiness just as much as you do. Maybe you can find a buddy to take on the 28-Day Revolution with you. Having the right friend to motivate and support you along the way can make all the difference. Sharing your progress through social media is a great way to pull in support from friends and family. If you're sharing your revolution on Instagram, make sure to tag me @dr.alandesmond and I'll help cheer you along the way.

PREP YOUR MICROBIOME

Your microbiome is in for a treat. During the 28-Day Revolution you'll achieve an impressive plant diversity, hitting between 50 and 70 unique plants per week! A significant increase in plant diversity and fibre might take your microbes and digestive system by surprise, leading to temporary feelings of digestive discomfort. And don't forget that a higher fibre diet leads to more trips to the bathroom!

If you have a history of avoiding fruits, vegetable and wholegrains, it's a good idea to increase the plants in your diet over a period of three to four weeks before embarking on the 28-Day Revolution. Start with breakfast, choosing a bowl of Perfect Porridge (page 64), Quick banana & blueberry pancakes (page 80) or any of the breakfast recipes to start your day. After two weeks, add some of the main meals and lighter meals, while making sure to snack on fresh fruit throughout the day. This will give your gut microbiome time to adjust to your new, healthier approach to food. When about half of the meals you eat in a week are plant-powered, you are ready for the 28-Day Revolution!

TIPS FOR EATING OUT

Most restaurants are now more than happy to cater for customers who prefer meals that are 100% plant-based. If you're dining out, you might like to call ahead and check. In my experience, if you ask the server or kitchen staff to recommend their healthiest vegan meal, they will be delighted to help. Just explain that you'd prefer a plant-based option that is also low in added oils (and not too sweet). If you're invited for dinner at a friend's house, why not volunteer to bring along some tempting plant-based dishes for everyone to try?

Remember: There is no such thing as perfection. If an occasional break from the plan helps you to get across the finish line, that is absolutely fine. Don't let the pursuit of perfection become the enemy of progress!

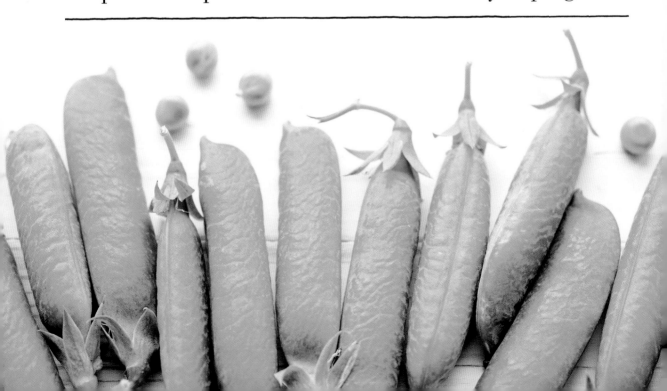

THE 28-DAY REVOLUTION:
LETTER FOR YOUR DOCTOR OR HEALTH PROFESSIONAL

Dear Doctor or Health Professional,

Your patient is embarking on the 28-Day Revolution, a four-week programme of eating healthy, plant-based meals. The recipes are firmly focused on wholefoods, with very little added salt or oil. The meal plans provide only healthy plant-based recipes, meaning that participants will not be eating eggs, dairy or meat products. They will be enjoying an extremely healthy version of an ideal Mediterranean diet.

Multiple medical studies have shown that this type of diet can be extremely effective in achieving healthy weight loss and improving markers of cardiovascular and overall health. Both the British Dietetic Association and the US Academy of Nutrition and Dietetics endorse a completely plant-based diet as being nutritionally adequate with wide-reaching health benefits at all stages of life.

The recipes and meal plans have been reviewed and approved by a registered dietitian. There is no calorie counting and no portion control. Participants are advised to eat according to their appetite. We also advise all participants to take a daily VEG-1 multivitamin, or equivalent, to ensure that they are getting enough of vitamins B12 and D3. Vitamin B12 supplementation is especially important if they decide to remain on a healthy plant-based diet in the long term.

Individuals on medication for high blood pressure
A healthy, whole-food diet with little added salt or oil can lead to improved control of high blood pressure. For this reason, individuals taking medication for hypertension are likely to see their blood pressure improve and it may even become low. For this reason, we advise obtaining a home blood pressure monitor and using it to monitor blood pressure at least once per day. Any person who experiences dizziness or faint episodes should see their GP or practice nurse as a matter of urgency.

Individuals on medication for type 2 diabetes
A healthy, whole-food diet without processed carbohydrates, meat or dairy can increase insulin sensitivity and lead to better control of blood sugars in individuals with type 2 diabetes. However, if participants are on medications to keep their blood sugars under control, they might notice that their blood sugars are running lower than usual and need to adjust their medications accordingly. This is especially important for those who take any form of insulin. We therefore advise any participants with diabetes to check their blood sugars regularly each day. Patients should always work with their usual doctor, nurse or dietitian while making these healthy changes to their diet and lifestyle.

The 28-Day Revolution is designed to be educational and evidence-based. Thank you so much for supporting your patient while they embark on this healthy lifestyle change.

With best wishes,

Dr Alan Desmond
Consultant Gastroenterologist & General Physician
For more information visit alandesmond.com/revolution

START THE REVOLUTION: MEAL PLANS & COOKING GUIDE

In this section you will find meal plans and lists of everything you need to shop for and cook during the 28-Day Revolution. Let's start with some tips and important points to bear in mind.

• The meal plans and shopping lists provide everything you need to prepare delicious, plant-based meals for 28 days. We've included breakfast, lunch, a main meal and a sweet treat. In between meals, please snack on three pieces of fruit per day, whichever ones you prefer. A fresh apple, a banana and an orange will do fine.

• Thanks to some strategic batch cooking and clever prep work, you'll be cooking on just four days of the week. If you need to take lunch to work, make it the night before and refrigerate in your lunchbox.

• Plan ahead. Some recipes need a little bit of prep work the day before. This is all laid out clearly in the step-by-step cooking guide. Having your ingredients ready to go in advance is a real time-saver.

• Store salad dressings and added garnishes in separate containers. Its best to add them to the dish just before serving.

• If you aren't used to having a lot of fresh veg in your cooking, this is the element that will initially slow down your meal prep. Don't allow this to stress you out. You'll get faster and more efficient with each day. By week three, you'll feel more at ease and efficient in your busy kitchen.

• When storing meals that are cooked ahead of time, cool the food quickly and thoroughly, perhaps by spreading it out on a plate or baking tray. Aim to refrigerate food within an hour. Transfer it to airtight containers and store in the fridge. Food should never be left out overnight.

• When reheating meals, ensure that everything is completely heated through and piping hot.

• Above all, have fun and enjoy the process. The time you spend in the kitchen will be an incredible investment in your health and well-being.

STORE-CUPBOARD SHOPPING LIST

These essentials set you up with all the store-cupboard goods needed to last you through the entire 28-Day Revolution. You'll find a separate shopping list of the fresh ingredients needed at the start of each week.

BEANS & PULSES

Black beans, 2 x 400g (14oz) cans
Black-eyed beans, 1 x 400g (14oz) can
Butter beans, 1 x 400g (14oz) can
Cannellini beans, 2 x 400g (14oz) cans
Chickpeas, 8 x 400g (14oz) cans
Cooked Puy lentils, 2 x 400g (14oz) cans
Haricot beans, 1 x 400g (14oz) can
Kidney beans, 1 x 400g (14oz) can
Red lentils, dried 200g (7oz)
Tempeh, 200g (7oz)
Tofu, firm or extra firm, 1kg (2¼lb)

PRESERVES, PICKLES & OTHER CANS

Capers, 1 x 200g (7oz) jar
Chopped tomatoes, 6 x 400g (14oz) cans
Green olives, 200g (7oz)
Half-fat coconut milk, 200ml (7oz)
Passata, 1 x 500ml (17fl oz) jar
Pitted black olives, 100g (4oz)
Preserved artichoke hearts, 1 x 280g (10oz) jar
Preserved lemons, 1 x 220g (7½oz) jar (optional)
Roasted & skinned red peppers, 2 x 350g (12oz) jars
Sauerkraut, 1 x 400g (14oz) jar

FROZEN FOOD

Frozen broad beans, 200g (7oz)
Frozen peas, 500g (18oz)

DRIED FRUIT & BAKING ITEMS

Baking powder
Bicarbonate of soda
Cacao nibs, 100g (4oz)
Cacao powder, 250g (8oz)
Cornflour, 1 packet
Dried apricots, 200g (7oz)
Dried sour cherries, 50g (2oz)
Maple syrup, 500ml (17fl oz)
Medjool dates, 500g (17oz)
Vanilla extract, 1 small bottle

DRIED HERBS & SPICES

Sea salt, 1 x 200g (7oz) tub
Black peppercorns in a grinder
Small jars of the following: allspice, bay leaves, caraway seeds, cardamom pods, cayenne pepper, chilli flakes, chilli powder, ground cinnamon, coriander and cumin, dried thyme, fennel seeds, garam masala, ground ginger, jerk seasoning, medium curry powder, nutmeg, oregano, saffron, sesame seeds, star anise, sweet smoked paprika, ground turmeric.

BEVERAGES

Coffee, 1 bag/jar
Red wine, 1 x 187ml (6½fl oz) bottle

NUTS & SEEDS

Almonds, flaked & toasted, 150g (5oz)
Almonds, ground, 50g (2oz)
Black onion seeds, 25g (1oz)
Cashew nuts, 100g (4oz)
Cooked chestnuts, 100g (4oz)
Hazelnuts, 150g (5oz)
Nut butter, 340g (12oz) jars x2
Peanuts, 50g (2oz)
Pine nuts, 50g (2oz)
Pistachios, 50g (2oz)
Pumpkin seeds, 50g (2oz)
Sunflower seeds, 50g (2oz)
Tahini, 1 x 300g (11oz) jar
Walnuts, 250g (9oz)

VINEGARS & OIL

(1 average bottle of each, unless specified otherwise)
Balsamic vinegar
Cider vinegar
Red wine vinegar
Rice vinegar
Extra virgin olive oil, 1 litre (2 pints)

WHOLEGRAINS

Brown basmati rice, 1kg (2¼lb)
Buckwheat flour, 200g (7oz)
Buckwheat noodles,100g (4oz)
Chickpea (gram) flour, 200g (7oz)
Cracked freekeh, 200g (7oz)
Farro, 100g (4oz)
Porridge oats, 1 kg (2¼lb)
Polenta, quick-cooking, 100g (4oz)
Quinoa, 300g (11oz)
Shell-like pasta, 500g (18oz)
Wholegrain spelt, 200g (7oz)
Wholemeal couscous, 100g (4oz)
Wholemeal flour, 500g (18oz)
Wholemeal spaghetti, 100g (4oz)
Wholemeal spelt flour, 200g (7oz)
Wild rice, 200g (7oz)

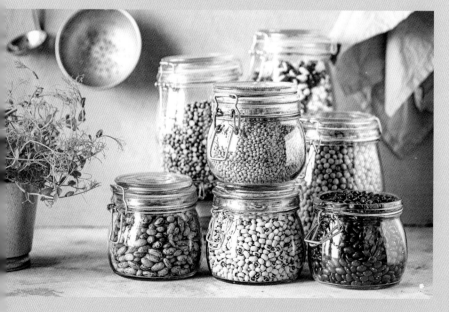

WEEK 1

DON'T FEEL HUNGRY

As you head into week 1 you might be feeling uncertain about how much food to eat. Don't worry! Since your meals will be naturally nutrient-dense rather than high-calorie, you have permission to eat a greater volume of food than you might be used to. Everyone is different. Listen to your natural appetite. If you're an active person, or if you're simply feeling hungry, here are a few ideas.

Don't be afraid to enjoy extra snacks if you feel like you need them. A slice of oat bread with a dollop of nut butter, an extra bowl of Simple Porridge, or a cup of Dreamy Hot Chocolate will give you the fuel needed to keep going between meals.

Bulk out any dish by adding a portion of sweet potato or brown rice to your plate. These whole carbohydrates promote feelings of fullness and better blood sugar control.

Feel free to mix it up. If you don't fancy the suggested meal plan, just dip into any of the other recipes. There are plenty more to explore.

Add a fourth meal to your day. Cook an extra portion, try one of the off-plan recipes, or use some leftovers from your meal prep.

The portion sizes allowed on the eating plans are generous. If you have a naturally smaller appetite, you might find that cooking just three times a week provides more than enough food for the whole week. If stored in an airtight container, your meals will keep just fine in the fridge for three or four days.

WEEK 1 SHOPPING LIST

Here are the fresh ingredients required for your first seven days

VEGETABLES
Asparagus, 200g (7oz)
Baby spinach, 150g (5oz)
Beetroot, 300g (11oz)
Butternut squash, 1 large
Carrots, 400g (14oz)
Celery, 1 head (should last you into week 2)
Cherry tomatoes, 400g (14oz)
Cucumber, 1
Fennel bulb, 1
Mixed summer berries, 150g (5oz)
New potatoes, 400g (14oz)
Radicchio or bitter leaves, 80g (3¼oz)
Red cabbage, 1 small head
Red onions, 4
Salad leaves, mixed, 100g (4oz)
Sweet potatoes, 600g (21oz)
Tomatoes, 2

FRUIT
Apples, 6
Bananas, 1 bunch of five
Lemons, 5
Lime, 1
Plus a selection of extra fruit for snacking – 3 items a day – apples, bananas, oranges or any of your favourite fruits

HERBS & FLAVOURINGS
Coriander, 60g (2¼oz)
Garlic, 2 bulbs
Mint leaves, 30g (about 1oz)
Parsley, 60g (2¼oz)

STORE-CUPBOARD PERISHABLES
Hummus, 1 x 200g (7oz) tub
Oat milk, 500ml (17fl oz)
Rye bread, 1 small loaf
Soya yogurt, 1 x 125g (4½oz) tub
Wholemeal bread, 1 small loaf
Wholemeal burger buns, 2
Wholemeal pittas, 2

MEAL PLAN

	MONDAY	TUESDAY	WEDNESDAY	THURSDAY	FRIDAY	SATURDAY	SUNDAY
BREAKFAST	Berry oat smoothie (page 74)		Nut butter & banana on toast (page 72) + 1 extra piece of fruit		Spelt & buckwheat pancakes (page 80) with stewed apples		Spring tofu hash (page 76)
LUNCH	MLT sandwich (page 98)		Wild rice super salad (page 116)		Speedy falafels (page 107) served with wraps, salad leaves, tomato and a half of the tahini dressing		Sweet potato with jerk black beans (page 87)
DINNER	Spanish rice with fennel, tomato & olives (page 156)		Pakora bean burgers with raita & sweet potato chips (page 162)		Squash & olive tagine with freekeh (page 148)		Epic Nut roast & onion miso gravy (page 166)
SNACKS & SWEET TREATS	Three pieces of fresh fruit and a Carrot cake bite (page 180) each day						

STEP-BY-STEP COOKING GUIDE

All the recipes make 2 portions – one to eat, and the other to keep for the following day. Just 1 portion of each meal is required on Sundays, so simply halve the ingredient amounts in the recipes.

SUNDAY EVENING

Prep for tomorrow: Put your smoothie oats together and leave to soak overnight. Make a batch of Carrot cake bites, then cool and cut them into at least 7 pieces. Finally, cook and cool the mushrooms for your MLT sandwich. Store everything in airtight containers in the fridge.

MONDAY

Breakfast: Blitz your Berry oats smoothie. Half is your breakfast. Keep the other half in an airtight container or bottle for breakfast tomorrow.
Lunch: Using your pre-cooked mushrooms, build an MLT sandwich.
Dinner: Make the Spanish rice with fennel, tomato & olives. Eat one portion for dinner. Cool and store the remainder for tomorrow.

TUESDAY

Breakfast: Drink your Berry oats smoothie after giving it a good shake or stir.
Lunch: Using your pre-cooked mushrooms, build an MLT sandwich.
Dinner: Reheat the Spanish rice leftovers. You might need to add a dash of hot water to help it along. Garnish and serve.

WEDNESDAY

Breakfast: Make your Nut butter & banana on toast. Enjoy it with an extra piece of fruit.
Lunch: Cook and cool the rice for the Wild rice salad. Slice the veg but don't dress them yet. When you're ready for lunch, mix a half portion of the salad with the dressing. Keep the other half separately in the fridge for tomorrow.
Dinner: Make the Pakora bean burger mix and keep half for tomorrow. Cook one burger and roast 1 serving of Sweet potato chips (they are best made fresh but can be reheated). Build your burger and serve with the chips.

THURSDAY

Breakfast: Make your Nut butter & banana on toast. Enjoy it with an extra piece of fruit.
Lunch: Dress the veggies remaining from yesterday and leave for 15 minutes or so. Add them to the remaining Wild rice salad along with the garnishes.
Dinner: Cook the Bean burger reserved from yesterday and make a fresh serving of Sweet potato chips. Eat them together.

FRIDAY

Breakfast: Make the Spelt & buckwheat pancake batter and the stewed apples. Use half the batter to make 4 pancakes and serve them with half the apples. Save the rest for Saturday.

Lunch: Make your Speedy falafels. Cook half of them and eat in a wholegrain pitta with tomato, salad leaves and half the tahini dressing. Put the other half in the fridge for tomorrow. (You could cook all the falafels today if you prefer because they can be eaten cold or reheated tomorrow.)
Dinner: Make the Squash & olive tagine. Eat half and cool the rest for tomorrow. The freekeh is best cooked and eaten fresh, so make a single serving today and cook a fresh serving tomorrow.

SATURDAY

Breakfast: Use the reserved Spelt & buckwheat batter to make 4 pancakes; serve with the remaining stewed apples.
Lunch: Cook (or reheat) the remaining Falafels and eat in a wholegrain pitta with tomato, salad leaves and the remaining tahini dressing.
Dinner: Put a portion of freekeh on to cook. Reheat the rest of the tagine. Finish the freekeh with the harissa and herbs.

SUNDAY

Cook the recipes for today at your leisure, using just half quantities, as you need only enough for one day.

WEEK 2

SHARE YOUR FOOD

You've learned so much over the past week about cooking exciting plant-based meals. Now is the perfect time to share your skills, so why not cook extra and invite a friend or family member to share a healthy plant-based meal? Once they've enjoyed a plate of Savoury farinata with courgettes, tomatoes & capers followed by a generous scoop of Banana pecan ice cream, they'll understand why you can't stop talking about this food. They might even want to start a plant-based revolution of their own!

If it's not practical to invite someone over, please share a photo of your food with me on Instagram. Tag me @dr.alandesmond and I'll let you know how impressed I am with your kitchen skills.

WEEK 2 SHOPPING LIST

Here are the fresh ingredients required for the next seven days.

VEGETABLES
Asparagus, 100g (4oz)
Aubergines, 2
Avocados, 3
Black kale, 150g (5oz)
Butternut squash, 1
Carrots, 1
Cauliflower, 1
Chard, 100g (4oz)
Cherry tomatoes, 400g (14oz)
Courgettes, 3
Mangetout, 50g (2oz)
Onions, 2
Pak choi, 1
Potatoes, 800g (2lb)
Radishes, 1 large bunch
Red onions, 2
Red peppers, 2
Spring greens, 300g (11oz)
Spring onions, 1 large bunch

Sprouted seeds or beans, 30g (about 1oz)
Sweetcorn cob, 1
Watercress, 50g (2oz)

FRUIT
Apples, 6
Bananas, 4
Blackberries, 100g (4oz)
Blueberries, 150g (5oz)
Lemons, 3
Lime, 1
Mango, 1
Passion fruit,1
Plus a selection of fruit for snacking – 3 pieces a day

HERBS & FLAVOURINGS
Basil, 20g (about 1oz)
Coriander, 40g (1½oz)
Garlic, 2 bulbs
Ginger, fresh root, 100g (4oz)
Mint leaves, 20g (about 1oz)
Red chillies, 3
Thyme leaves, 10g (about ½oz)

STORE-CUPBOARD PERISHABLES
Almond milk, 500ml (17fl oz)
Coconut milk (drinking), 350ml (12fl oz)
Oat milk, 500ml (17fl oz)
Rye bread, 1small loaf
Wholemeal bread, 1 small loaf

MEAL PLAN

	MONDAY	TUESDAY	WEDNESDAY	THURSDAY	FRIDAY	SATURDAY	SUNDAY
BREAKFAST	Quinoa porridge with blackberries & pistachios (page 64)		Nut butter & banana on toast (page 72) plus 1 extra piece of fruit		Tropical oats smoothie (page 75)		Quick banana & blueberry pancakes (page 80)
LUNCH	Fiery noodle salad (page 96)		Chunky minestrone (page 108)		Savoury farinata with courgettes, tomatoes & capers (page 92)		Avocado on toast with radishes (page 118)
DINNER	Goulash hotpot (page 160)		Cauliflower, butter bean & chard dhal (page 154)		Corn, & squash spelt risotto with black kale (page 128)		Miso aubergines with tofu fried rice (page 168)
SNACKS & SWEET TREATS	3 pieces of fresh fruit each day + a portion of Apple and apricot crumble (page 182)				3 pieces of fresh fruit every day + a mug of Dreamy hot chocolate (page 180)		

STEP-BY-STEP COOKING GUIDE

MONDAY

Breakfast: The Quinoa porridge is so simple and quick to make that you needn't prepare it in advance. Cook half the amounts listed to make one serving.
Lunch: Cook and cool the noodles for the Fiery noodle salad. Slice the veg and make the dressing. Mix half together for your lunch. Store the remaining prepped ingredients separately in the fridge for tomorrow.
Dinner: Make the Goulash hotpot. Eat half and cool the other half for tomorrow. Cook only one serving of greens for tonight; tomorrow's are best cooked fresh.

TUESDAY

Breakfast: Cook half the amounts listed for Quinoa porridge to make one serving.
Lunch: Mix the remaining noodles, veg and dressing together for your Fiery noodle salad.
Dinner: Cover the remaining Goulash hotpot with foil and place in an oven preheated to 180°C/Fan 160°C/350°F/Gas 4 for about 25 minutes, or until piping hot. Remove the foil for the final 5 minutes to re-crisp the topping. Cook a fresh serving of greens to go alongside.

WEDNESDAY

Breakfast: Make your Nut butter & banana on toast. Eat some fresh fruit alongside it.
Lunch: Make the Chunky minestrone soup. Eat half and cool the other half for tomorrow.
Dinner: Make the Cauliflower, butter bean & chard dahl. Eat half and cool the rest for tomorrow.

THURSDAY

Breakfast: Make your Nut butter & banana on toast. Eat with an extra piece of fresh fruit.
Lunch: Reheat your leftover Chunky minestrone.
Dinner: Reheat your Cauliflower, butter bean & chard dahl.
Prep for breakfast: Put the Tropical oats smoothie together and leave to soak overnight.

FRIDAY

Breakfast: Blitz your Tropical oats smoothie. Eat half and store the remainder in an airtight container for tomorrow.
Lunch: Make the Savoury farinata and filling. Eat half and cool the rest for tomorrow.
Dinner: Make the Corn & squash spelt risotto. Eat half and cool the rest for tomorrow.

SATURDAY

Breakfast: Enjoy the remaining portion of your Tropical oats smoothie.
Lunch: Reheat the remaining Farinata and filling separately in a non-stick frying pan or hot oven. Serve together.
Dinner: Reheat the leftover Risotto on the hob, adding a dash of hot water or stock to prevent it sticking to the pan.

SUNDAY

Cook today's recipes, using half the amounts listed, as you only need enough for today.
Prep for next week: Make a batch of Cherry cacao bars. Once cooled and cut into pieces (at least one for each day), store in an airtight container.

WEEK 3

YOU CAN DO THIS

Let's start this week with a strong, positive focus on the reasons why you decided to change the food on your plate. Whatever goals you set yourself as you embarked on this plant-based adventure, you are three weeks closer to achieving them. It's likely that you've already experienced benefits that you never expected. Have you noticed increased energy levels? Improved quality of sleep? An increased feeling of well-being? This is what life feels like as you thrive on the simple wholefoods that have nourished humans for generations. Keep going. You can do this!

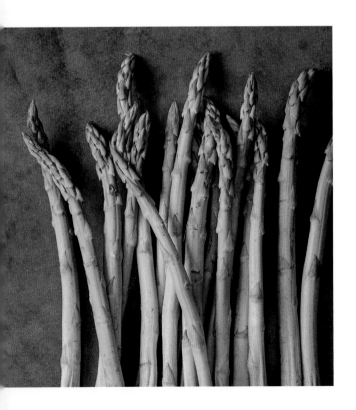

WEEK 3 SHOPPING LIST

The fresh ingredients required for the next seven days.

VEGETABLES
Asparagus, 150g (5oz)
Black kale, 150g (5oz)
Carrots, 1
Celeriac, 1
Celery, 1 head
Cooked beetroot, 150g (5oz)
Courgette, 1
Cucumber, 1
Fennel bulb, 1
French beans, 100g (4oz)
Green cabbage, 1 small head
Mushrooms, chestnut, 100g (4oz)
Onions, 1
Portobello mushrooms, 200g (7oz)
Potatoes, 1
Red onions, 2
Red peppers, 1
Spring onions, 3
Sweet potatoes, 150g (5oz)
Tomatoes, 2

FRUIT
Bananas, 3
Blueberries, 150g (5oz)
Lemon, 1
Strawberries, 400g
Plus a selection of fruit for snacking – 3 items a day

HERBS & FLAVOURINGS
Basil, 40g (1½oz)
Coriander, 20g (¾oz)
Dill, 20g (¾oz)
Garlic bulbs, 2
Parsley, 60g (1½oz)
Rosemary, 20g (¾oz)

STORE-CUPBOARD PERISHABLES
Wholemeal bread, 1 loaf
Oat milk, 600ml (1 pint)
Rye bread, 1 small loaf

MEAL PLAN

	MONDAY	TUESDAY	WEDNESDAY	THURSDAY	FRIDAY	SATURDAY	SUNDAY
BREAKFAST	Simple oat porridge (page 64) + strawberries, blueberries or raspberries		Nut butter & banana on toast (page 72) + 1 extra piece of fruit		Quick banana & blueberry pancakes (page 80)		Spicy baked beans with sweet potato farls (page 78)
LUNCH	Beetroot, sauerkraut & watercress sandwich (page 100)		Squash & raw kale quinoa salad (page 114)		Spanish red pepper soup (page 110)		Avocado on toast with miso 'shrooms (page 190)
DINNER	Sweet potato Massaman curry (page 152)		Summer veg & white bean pasta (page 140)		Rosti pie with braised cabbage & peas (page 126)		Stuffed peppers with artichokes, fennel & farro (page 138)
SNACKS & SWEET TREATS	Three pieces of fresh fruit and a Cherry cacao bar (page 192) each day						

STEP-BY-STEP COOKING GUIDE

MONDAY

Breakfast: Cook 1 portion of Simple oat porridge and top with fresh berries of your choice.

Lunch: Make the full amount of filling for the Beetroot, sauerkraut & watercress sandwich, but use only half today; save the rest for tomorrow.

Dinner: Make the Sweet potato Massaman curry, saving half for tomorrow. Cook just the amount of rice (75g) you need for today, as it is safer to cook rice as required than to reheat it.

TUESDAY

Breakfast: Cook 1 portion of Simple oat porridge and serve with fresh berries.

Lunch: Use the remaining beetroot filling to build a sandwich.

Dinner: Reheat the Sweet potato curry and cook a fresh portion of rice to go with it.

Prep for tomorrow: Cover 50g (2oz) cashew nuts with water and leave in the fridge to soak (they are needed for the dressing that goes with the squash salad).

WEDNESDAY

Breakfast: Make your Nut butter & banana on toast. Eat some fresh fruit alongside it.

Lunch: Prepare the Squash & raw kale quinoa salad, keeping the kale separate. Set half aside to cool and store for tomorrow. Combine today's portion with half the kale and the cashew dressing, saving the rest for tomorrow.

Dinner: Make the sauce for the Summer veg & white bean pasta and reserve half for tomorrow. The garnish and the pasta are best made freshly as needed, so just make half the amount for today.

THURSDAY

Breakfast: Make your Nut butter & banana on toast. Eat with an extra piece of fresh fruit.

Lunch: Toss all the remaining Squash salad ingredients together and add the cashew dressing.

Dinner: Reheat the Summer veg pasta sauce. Cook a fresh portion of pasta and make a fresh batch of garnish.

FRIDAY

Breakfast: Make the Banana and blueberry pancake batter. Use half now to make 4 pancakes, and keep the remainder in the fridge for tomorrow.

Lunch: Make the Spanish red pepper soup. Eat half now and cool the remainder for tomorrow.

Dinner: Make the Rosti pie. Eat half now and cool the remainder for tomorrow. Cook just half the amounts of cabbage and peas as they are best cooked fresh each day.

SATURDAY

Breakfast: Use the remaining Banana & blueberry batter to make 4 pancakes.

Lunch: Reheat your remaining Spanish red pepper soup.

Dinner: Cover the remaining Rosti pie with foil and place in an oven preheated to 180°C/Fan 160°C/350°F/Gas 4 for about 25 minutes, or until piping hot. Remove the foil for the final 5 minutes to re-crisp the topping. Cook a fresh serving of cabbage and peas to serve alongside.

SUNDAY

Cook the recipes for today at your leisure, halving the amounts as you only need enough for today.

Prep for next week: Put the Mocha oats ingredients together to soak overnight. Make a batch of Beanie brownies, keeping half in the fridge and freezing the other half for later in the week. Remember to defrost them a day before needed. If you like, they can be warmed up for 8-10 minutes in an oven preheated to 180°C/Fan 160°C/350°F/Gas 4.

WEEK 4

KEEP LEARNING

Throughout this book I've shared the science that has shaped my medical practice and detailed exactly how a plant-based diet can transform your health. As you get ready to cross the finishing line on the 28-Day Revolution you may be thinking about life after these four weeks. This is a great time to take your plant-based education to the next level. Whether you prefer listening to podcasts, reading books by other plant-based doctors and chefs, watching full-length documentaries or shorter educational videos, you'll find a list of fantastic resources to help you continue your learning journey on page 218.

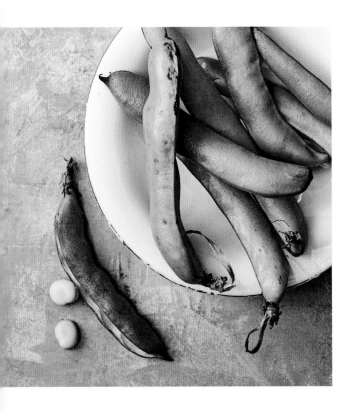

WEEK 4 SHOPPING LIST

The fresh ingredients required for the next seven days.

VEGETABLES
Aubergine, 1
Avocado, 2
Baby spinach, 150g (5oz)
Butternut squash, 1
Carrots, 2
Chestnut mushrooms, 100g (4oz)
Cucumber, 1
Leek, 1
Little gem lettuce, 1
Parsnips, 300g (11oz)
Portobello mushrooms, 2
Radishes, small bunch (about 200g/7oz)
Red onions, 5
Red peppers, 2
Salad leaves, 50g (2oz)
Spring onions, small bunch (about 100g/4oz)
Sweet potatoes, 2
Tomatoes, 7

FRUIT
Apples, 3
Bananas, 5
Blueberries, 200g (7oz)
Lemons, 6
Limes, 2
Plus a selection of fruit for snacking – 3 items a day

HERBS & FLAVOURINGS
Coriander, 60g (2½oz)
Garlic bulbs, 2
Ginger, fresh root 100g (4oz)
Mint leaves, 20g (about 1oz)
Parsley, 100g (4oz)
Red chilli, 1
Rosemary leaves, 20g (about 1oz)

STORE-CUPBOARD PERISHABLES
Oat milk, 400ml (14fl oz)
Rye bread, 1 small loaf
Wholegrain baguette rolls, 2
Wholemeal tortillas, 2

MEAL PLAN	MONDAY	TUESDAY	WEDNESDAY	THURSDAY	FRIDAY	SATURDAY	SUNDAY
BREAKFAST	Mocha oat smoothie (page 74)		Nut butter & banana on toast (page 72) + 1 extra piece of fruit		Spelt & buckwheat pancakes (page 80) with blueberries		Kedgeree with roast tomatoes, mushrooms & spinach (page 82)
LUNCH	Speedy falafels (page 107) with tahini sauce (page 132)		Spicy parsnip & lentil winter soup (page 112)		Spicy tofu rolls (page 102)		Sweet potato with chickpea tabbouleh (page 86)
DINNER	Hearty Bolognese with squash & rosemary polenta (page 124)		One-pot chilli bowl (page 164)		Plant-powered stew with braised chickpeas & couscous (page 134)		Crispy tofu tacos & chopped salsa salad (page 130)
SNACKS & SWEET TREATS	Three pieces of fresh fruit and a Beanie brownie (page 184) each day						

STEP-BY-STEP COOKING GUIDE

MONDAY

Breakfast: Blitz the Mocha oat smoothie. Have half today and store the remainder in an airtight container for tomorrow.

Lunch: Make the Speedy falafels and cook just half of them, saving the rest for tomorrow. Serve in a pitta bread with sliced tomato, salad leaves and half the tahini sauce, saving the rest for tomorrow.

Dinner: Make the Hearty Bolognese & polenta. Eat half, then cool and store the remainder in the fridge for tomorrow.

TUESDAY

Breakfast: Shake or stir the remaining Mocha oat smoothie before drinking.

Lunch: Cook the remaining falafels and eat them in a pitta bread with sliced tomato, salad leaves and the remaining tahini dressing.

Dinner: Reheat the Hearty Bolognese & polenta. If reheating in a pan, watch to make sure that the polenta doesn't burn.

WEDNESDAY

Breakfast: Make your Nut butter & banana on toast. Serve with an extra piece of fresh fruit.

Lunch: Make the Spicy parsnip & lentil soup. Eat half and cool the remainder for tomorrow.

Dinner: Cook the One-pot chilli. Eat half, topping it with half the garnish. Cool the remaining chilli and store in the fridge, along with the remaining garnish, for tomorrow.

THURSDAY

Breakfast: Make your Nut butter & banana on toast. Serve with an extra piece of fresh fruit.

Lunch: Reheat the remaining portion of Spicy parsnip & lentil soup.

Dinner: Reheat and garnish the remaining One-pot chilli.

Optional prep for tomorrow: Marinate, cook and cool the tofu for the Spicy tofu rolls, and make the pickled veg. Store in the fridge.

FRIDAY

Breakfast: Make the Spelt & buckwheat pancake batter. Use half to make 4 pancakes, and serve with blueberries. Save the remaining batter for tomorrow.

Lunch: Build your Spicy tofu rolls using half the ingredients you prepared the night before; the tofu can be reheated or used cold. If making the rolls fresh, reserve half the tofu and veg for Saturday. Fry the tofu and build your sandwich, adding half the pickled veg.

Dinner: Make the Plant-powered stew. Eat half, then cool and store the remainder for tomorrow.

SATURDAY

Breakfast: Use the remaining batter to make 4 pancakes and serve them with blueberries.

Lunch: Make your Spicy tofu rolls with the ingredients you prepped earlier, or make them fresh with the reserved tofu and veg. The rolls are great served cold or reheated.

Dinner: Reheat the remaining Plant-powered stew.

SUNDAY

Cook the recipes for today at your leisure. Halve the amounts as you only need enough for today – unless you'd like to have delicious leftovers to start the rest of your plant-based adventures tomorrow!

CELEBRATE SUCCESS AND MOVE FORWARD

Congratulations! You have officially completed the 28-Day Revolution! Over the last 28 days you have prepped, chopped and cooked your way to better health. You've shown that you too can thrive on a whole-food, plant-based diet. As you look back at the goals you set for this challenge, I hope that you enjoy putting big tick marks next to many of them. They are no longer goals, they are now accomplishments. Take some time to celebrate your progress. Call the friends and family members who supported you on this 28-day journey and let them know that you just crossed the finish line in style. Get busy bragging about it on your social media – tag me on Instagram @dr.alandesmond and I'll send you a virtual high five. You did it!

By embracing the 28-Day Revolution, you made the decision to prioritise your health at every meal. Having discovered the powerful health benefits of a plant-fuelled gut microbiome, you have just achieved a plant diversity that is rarely seen in the 21st century. While others survive on foods that increase their risk of long-term illness and can take years off their natural life expectancy, you've chosen a different path – one that recognises food as the key to maximising your well-being and your chances of a long and vibrant life.

Throughout this book, I've shared the scientific evidence that has shaped my medical practice and transformed the lives of many of my patients. You've seen how joining the plant-based diet revolution can rapidly improve health and well-being and you've discovered the multiple benefits of a plant-fuelled gut microbiome. You've explored numerous studies revealing the true power of the food on your plate, with the ability to combat chronic inflammation, dramatically improve digestion, kickstart healthy weight loss, reverse insulin resistance, fight heart disease, and even to increase happiness and help to treat depression. All in a matter of weeks! By completing the 28-Day Revolution you may have experienced these immediate benefits for yourself. But we both know that the advantages of joining this revolution go way beyond 28 days.

I truly hope that today marks the beginning of a lifelong revolution in your approach to food. You have the knowledge, the recipes and the kitchen skills you need. Make sure to read Part 5, where you'll find some of my favourite cookbooks, answers to commonly asked questions and other valuable resources to help you continue on your plant-based journey successfully.

The evidence is clear. A whole-food, plant-based diet is the optimal diet for human health and longevity. The more plant-based the better. I truly hope that you've enjoyed The Plant-Based Diet Revolution. Choosing to continue your life fuelled exclusively by plants may prove to be the best decision you've ever made.

PART FIVE

QUESTIONS, ANSWERS & RECOMMENDED RESOURCES

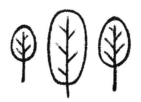

PLANT-BASED Q&A

Over the years I've offered support to thousands of people on the journey to a plant-based diet. Here are some practical and evidence-based answers to their most frequently asked questions.

Do you eat a plant-based diet?

Yes, I've eaten a whole-food and completely plant-based diet since 2016. My wife and children, and many of my friends and colleagues, also enjoy a plant-based diet and lifestyle. As a doctor who strongly recommends this approach to eating, I recognised years ago that this was the healthiest choice for me, my family and my patients.

Why don't your recipes include plant-based meats?

The recipes for the revolution make fruits, vegetables, beans, greens and wholegrains the stars of every meal. Enjoying a variety of these wholefoods is the key to unlocking the advantages of a plant-based diet. For this reason, the recipes avoid processed meat alternatives, which are often high in added saturated fats, salt and flavour enhancers. (362)

If you feel that the occasional plant-based sausage or meat-free burger helps you to keep on track, then please feel free to add them to any of our recipes. Although not wholefoods, they still have a lot of advantages to offer. They are free of harmful cholesterol and animal protein, and many even contain fibre. Make sure to check the label – ideally you want a product that is low in both salt and saturated fat.

Should I take an omega-3 oil supplement?

A plant-based diet has tremendous benefits to your health, but taking an omega-3 oil supplement might offer some additional advantages. Omega-3 fatty acids are among a group of healthy oils, also known as polyunsaturated fatty acids. They are important in maintaining the health of our heart, lungs, immune system and brain. There are two types: short-chain omega-3 (called ALA) and long-chain omega-3 (called EPA and DHEA).

Short-chain omega-3 is found in flaxseeds, chia seeds, walnuts, leafy green vegetables and soya beans. The body uses it to manufacture the long-chain omega-3s it needs. (363, 364) Many experts recommend getting additional long-chain omega-3s in your diet. One great source of EPA and DHEA are aquatic plants called algae. As fish eat a lot of algae, eating oily fish or taking a fish-oil supplement can tick the long-chain omega-3 box. However, you can get all your need by taking a daily 250–500mg of a plant-based omega-3 supplement. There are lots of brands available; most are made by extracting omega-3-rich oil directly from algae. As the algae are purpose-grown and harvested in clean water, these supplements have the added advantage of containing none of the heavy metals and other pollutants that come built in with fish and fish oils. (365, 366)

The science does not clearly show that people who eat a whole-food, plant-based diet get additional benefits from an omega-3 supplement, but many doctors and dietitians recommend it.

Are foods made from soya beans good for us?

Although the health benefits of beans are widely accepted, there is one bean that gets people worried. 'Is soya healthy?' is one of the most common questions I'm asked. There are many confusing and unfounded myths stating that soya beans are bad for your health. Beans and legumes in general have so many benefits that eating even small amounts each day can reduce blood pressure and prevent heart disease. Soya beans have added benefits, including healthy polyunsaturated oils and anti-oestrogenic effects, which protect against breast and prostate cancer. (367) Foods made from soya beans, such as tempeh and tofu, have been staples in Asia for centuries and are now firmly established globally. Even my small local supermarket now stocks a range of tofus and a UK-made organic tempeh.

Soya beans are also a nice way to increase the diversity of plants in your diet and promote beneficial changes in your gut microbiome. The fibre and fermentable carbohydrates in tofu work as prebiotics, feeding your healthy gut bugs and reducing the number of harmful ones. Fermented soy foods such as tempeh may be even more beneficial, adding ready-made fibre-loving bacteria to our microbial mix. (368)

Should I avoid gluten?

Gluten is a plant protein. It occurs naturally in wholegrains, including wheat, rye, barley and spelt. It's a stretchy protein, which makes it useful in giving breads, cakes and doughs their pleasant soft texture. Regular wholegrain consumption is one of the hallmarks of a healthy diet. (369) However, there are a few specific conditions where gluten-containing wholegrains might need to be avoided:

Coeliac disease is an auto-immune condition that affects about 1 in 100 people. It causes gut inflammation that usually heals completely on a healthy, gluten-free diet. (370) If you suspect that you may have coeliac disease, please ask your GP for a blood test to check for this diagnosis before you choose to go gluten-free.

Non-coeliac wheat sensitivity is a diagnosis made in people who have gut symptoms provoked by wheat, but test negative for coeliac disease. (371) It's thought to be rare and can be difficult to diagnose. In my experience, patients who suspect that they have this condition generally tolerate wholegrains just fine once they have improved the overall quality of their diet.

People with a *true wheat allergy* may have mild symptoms, but some can become seriously unwell, with difficulty breathing and anaphylaxis. The reaction is provoked by an allergy to gluten or to one of the other proteins found in wheat. It's diagnosed by testing the blood for a specific antibody and usually requires the input of a doctor with expertise in disorders of the immune system. (372) Individuals with a serious wheat allergy must be extremely cautious to avoid significant exposure and are advised to keep an epinephrine injection (or EpiPen) with them at all times.

Taken in combination, these three conditions probably affect fewer than 2% of the population. For everybody else, wholegrains and gluten should be on the menu. If you have had medical advice to avoid gluten entirely, please ask your doctor or dietitian if naturally gluten-free wholegrains, such as rice, buckwheat, millet, oats and sorghum, are suitable for you.

Is coffee a healthy choice?

Coffee is one of my favourite plants. While a regular cup of the black stuff was once regarded as the hallmark of an unhealthy lifestyle, in recent years scientists have woken up to its benefits. Drinking three cups a day is associated with multiple benefits: 19% reduction in death due to cardiovascular disease; 30% reduction in death due to stroke; 18% reduction in cancer, particularly cancers of the prostate, uterus and mouth, and melanoma and leukaemia. (373) A minor coffee addiction seems particularly beneficial in terms of gut health, and is associated with significant reductions in liver cirrhosis, liver cancer and colon cancer. However, there are two groups who should keep their consumption below 1–2 mugs per day – pregnant women and those with osteoporosis.

The coffee bean undergoes a chemical transformation on its journey from plant to cup. The final chemical composition of the brew depends on bean variety, degree of roasting, grind setting and brew type. Every cup contains at least 1,000 bioactive chemicals, including caffeine, chlorogenic acids, cafestol and kahweol. Many of these have potential for antioxidant, ant-inflammatory or anti-cancer action, but more research is needed. Some people are sensitive to coffee's jittery side effects. If it reduces your sense of well-being, please stick to decaffeinated coffee and other beverages, while continuing to focus on the other health-promoting aspects of your diet and lifestyle. Various teas, especially green teas, are also packed with plant-derived compounds that have antioxidative, anti-inflammatory, antihypertensive and cholesterol-lowering properties. (391)

Doesn't milk build better bones?

Calcium is a soil mineral, which is absorbed by plants as they grow. When cows eat the plants, some of that calcium is secreted in their milk. Although cow's milk is often promoted to parents and schoolchildren as essential for stronger bones, consumption of milk during adolescence does not protect from fractures in adulthood. While three daily servings of dairy have been recommended for bone health, there is no convincing evidence to support this advice. (374-375) To maintain healthy bones, the World Health Organization recommends eating at least 500mg of calcium per day. (376) On a whole-food plant-based diet, calcium is quite difficult to avoid. Some of my favourite calcium-rich foods are tofu, leafy greens, kale, beans and nuts. The 28-Day Revolution meal plans provide an average of 780mg of calcium per day. People who need more than this - those with osteoporosis or who are breastfeeding, for example - can top up with the calcium-rich foods listed on page 17. It's also important to remember that bone health is about more than just calcium. Protein, potassium and magnesium all contribute to building better bones, and all are available in a plant-based diet. Getting enough vitamin D, not smoking and taking regular weight-bearing exercise are also important.

Will I get enough iron on a plant-based diet?

Just like calcium, iron is a soil mineral, and all the naturally occurring iron found in foods was originally extracted from the earth by plants. In the UK it is recommended that most adults have a dietary iron intake of 8.7mg per day. However, women between the ages of 19 and 50, should aim for a higher intake of 14.8mg per day. Iron is found in dozens of plants, but beans, tofu, lentils, chickpeas, flaxseeds, pumpkin seeds, kale, figs and raisins are particularly good sources. Boost iron absorption by including a source of vitamin C – such as broccoli, cabbage, sprouts or any fruit – with your meal. The 28-Day Revolution meal plans provide an average of 20mg of iron per day. By eating a plant-based diet with a firm focus on healthy wholefoods, you will easily exceed your daily iron needs. (377-380)

Is a plant-based diet healthy for children?

A plant-based diet is just as healthy for children as it is for adults. (381-383) According to the American Dietetic Association, plant-based diets 'satisfy nutrient needs of infants, children, and adolescents and promote normal growth'. The British Nutrition Federation has reassured parents that 'breastfed children born to vegan mothers and weaned onto a vegan diet grow and develop normally'. Being surrounded by healthier food choices at home helps to establish lifelong healthy eating patterns. Trying to get your children to eat the foods you'd like them to eat is different matter entirely! If you're raising children on a plant-based diet, please see the extremely useful resources at vegansociety.com/resources/nutrition-and-health/life-stages

Is a plant-based diet beneficial in pregnancy?

A plant-based diet is a healthy option at all life stages, including pregnancy and during breastfeeding. A healthy plant-based approach that includes fruits, vegetables, legumes and wholegrains may even bring a reduced risk of developing diabetes during pregnancy. All pregnant and breastfeeding women, including those eating a plant-based diet, need to take extra care to ensure that all their baby's nutritional needs are met. (382-384) You can download a comprehensive advice sheet on nutrition in pregnancy at vegansociety.com/resources/downloads/pregnancy-and-breastfeeding

Do I need to worry about 'plant lectins'?

Lectins are a family of proteins which are found in many foods, especially wholegrains and beans. In 2017 a best-selling book claimed that the lectins in these foods are bad for us. (385) The language used was vivid, warning that lectins 'incite a kind of chemical warfare in our bodies, causing inflammatory reactions that can lead to weight gain and serious health conditions'. I'm sure the author was well-motivated in publishing these theories, but the science does not add up. As we've discussed throughout this book; fruits, vegetables, wholegrains, beans and other legumes are main components of the meals enjoyed by the healthiest populations in the world. (386, 387)

There is a simple explanation. Experiments conducted in the lab have indeed shown that raw or uncooked lectins can bind to glucose receptors, insulin receptors, thyroid cells and pancreatic cells. But the small amounts of lectins found in certain fruits and vegetables are not toxic. Add to this the fact that lectins are destroyed by simply cooking your food in the normal fashion and it's easy to see why there is no real cause for concern. Cooked or canned beans and wholegrain breads contain zero or almost zero lectins. (388, 389) If you don't eat raw beans – and you shouldn't – then you don't need to worry about lectins.

Should I eat a low FODMAP diet?

FODMAPs stands for 'fermentable oligo-saccharides, di-saccharides, mono-saccharides and polyols'. (391) Sometimes referred to as 'fermentable carbohydrates', FODMAPs are generally beneficial and help our healthy gut bacteria to flourish. Wholegrains, garlic, onions, avocados, apples and mangoes are some of my favourite foods and they are all high in FODMAPs. However, for people with IBS-type symptoms, or those who experience a lot of bloating and gas on a whole-food, plant-based diet, going through the process of eliminating and then gradually reintroducing the foods that are high in FODMAPs can be really helpful.

A few years ago I teamed up with Stephen and David Flynn of The Happy Pear and registered dietitian Rosie Martin to design 'The Happy Gut Course' a whole-food, plant-based online course that does just that. It has been incredibly successful in helping people to improve their digestive health. If you'd like to learn more about going through the FODMAP process while maintaining a varied plant-based diet, visit www.alandesmond.com/happygut

Should I worry about choline deficiency?

In 2019, an opinion piece appeared in the *British Medical Journal*, claiming that eating a completely plant-based diet could put people at risk of not getting enough choline in their diet. (392) Choline is an essential nutrient, required for healthy liver function, brain function and for neurological development. The article also highlighted that meat and eggs contain significant amounts of choline, and might be able to prevent any health problems arising from 'choline deficiency'. Although this article made headlines the world over, it soon came to light that it was written by a nutritionist who was also a paid consultant for both the British meat and egg industries. (393-4)

Within weeks, a spokesperson for the British Dietetic Association issued a statement to reassure the public that 'you absolutely can meet the requirements with a vegan or plant-based diet'. (395) Why? Because choline is also found in beans, potatoes, chickpeas, soya beans, oats and many more plant-based foods. In fact, as discussed on pages 36 and 55, the excess choline and cholesterol found in animal products may be key drivers of heart disease and vascular dementia! So please don't worry about 'choline deficiency' while you enjoy all the benefits of your new, healthier approach to food.

THE A TO Z OF PLANTS IN YOUR KITCHEN

This book would never have happened without the tireless input of my friend and co-author, the extraordinarily talented chef Bob Andrew. From artichokes to zucchini, here are Bob's expert tips for getting the best from the plants in your kitchen.

ARTICHOKES are delicious but require a lot of preparation to trim down to the usable flesh. It is a skill worth acquiring, but you can buy them prepared and cooked in jars or at the deli. No one will judge you for it!

ASPARAGUS is an iconic spring veg and grows supremely well in the UK. Simply snap off the tough woody ends before cooking. The spears need only a light steam or boil, but will equally be happy roasted in a hot oven, griddled or barbecued.

AUBERGINES are phenomenally tasty when cooked well. The best method is to bake them whole until the flesh is completely soft and collapsing. When buying, look for a heavy tight-skinned specimen. If you've never cooked an aubergine before, try the plant-powered stew on page 134.

AVOCADOS are eaten raw and loved for their rich taste and creamy texture. Ripe ones 'give' to a moderate squeeze. If unripe, keep them at room temperature near a banana, as the ethylene gas from the banana helps them ripen. Once opened, carefully scoop out the stone with a teaspoon and add a squeeze of lemon or lime to stop the flesh browning.

BEANS AND LEGUMES are powerhouses of protein, complex carbohydrates and fibre. For convenience, we've used cooked and canned varieties in most of the recipes, but there's nothing to stop you cooking them yourself straight from the packet. Note that dried chickpeas and beans need to be soaked overnight, then drained and covered with fresh water to cook. (You can throw in some garlic, herbs and spices if you like.) Bring to the boil, then simmer for 45–60 minutes, or until completely tender. Drain and rinse before adding to a dish.

BRASSICAS include all forms of cabbage, including Savoy, red and pointed, but also Brussels sprouts, cauliflowers, broccoli and the increasingly popular kales and spring and summer greens. They can all be boiled, steamed, stir-fried and even roasted. Just take care not to overcook them, as this will release a sulphurous aroma. (Red cabbage and black kale don't have this problem.) Store these veg in the fridge.

CELERY can be eaten raw, but when cooked, it is almost as important as onion in adding flavour to soups and stews.

CHICKPEAS can be soaked and cooked from dry in the same way as split peas and lentils, but are much easier to buy ready-cooked and canned. They are the basis of hummus and can be added to any stew or curry for added plant-based protein. They also become wonderfully crisp if roasted.

CHILLIES impart a fresher and fruitier flavour when used fresh. Their heat is concentrated in the seeds, so remove them before chopping if you want a milder hit. While often cooked into a dish, chillies can be eaten raw in a salsa or as a garnish.

FRUIT (DRIED) has an intense sweetness that is great in breakfasts and desserts, but can also be useful in savoury dishes – perhaps adding texture to a salad, or sweetness to a spicy stew. Ideally, choose fruit that has been naturally dried without the use of sulphides; the colour might be duller (apricots, for example, will be dark brown rather than orange), but the taste will be better. Another tip – check the packaging and avoid those with added sugar, particularly mangoes, cherries and cranberries.

FRUIT (FRESH) can be both a great ingredient and the perfect snack food to enjoy throughout the day. In this book all the fruit mentioned in the recipes, except for rhubarb (which needs cooking and sweetening) can be used raw. Always try to buy fresh, seasonal fruit. Frozen fruit, especially frozen berries, will work fine in any of the recipes. Some fruit, e.g. lemons, apples and even cucumbers, are wax coated to extend their shelf life and give an attractive shine. Try to buy unwaxed or scrub the produce to remove the coating. Lemons, limes and oranges are invaluable for dressing and finishing dishes, as the sharpness gives a distinct lift.

FENNEL has an aniseed flavour that mellows when cooked. Use it raw in salads and slaws, or slow cooked in stews and soups. Keep the fronds for garnishing.

HERBS (DRIED) can be useful when fresh ones aren't available. Woody ones lend themselves better to drying and retain more of their character, so keep a small store of dried thyme, rosemary, oregano and bay leaves. With the possible exception of mint, the soft and grassy herbs are best used fresh.

HERBS (FRESH) should be bought in small amounts as and when you need them (or grow your own for extra fresh). Thyme, rosemary, bay, sage and oregano are examples of woody or hardy varieties, and these robust types readily impart their flavour and fragrance when cooked or used in marinades. However, they can often be too powerful to use raw in large amounts, and are sometimes removed from the dish before serving. Parsley, coriander, mint, dill and basil are examples of soft or grassy herbs, and their leaves are most often added at the end of a dish's cooking time as too much heat can rob them of their character and freshness. They are ideal as a garnish, or even thrown in with salad leaves to add interest. Although the key notes are distinct, they all bring a clean freshness to any dish.

GINGER ROOT has a warm, sweet and earthy taste. It even has a slight heat to it if used in large amounts. Although heavily associated with spice and curry, it also does well in sweet dishes. When buying, look for plump pieces with no obvious dehydration or withering. Before using, remove the skin with the tip of a teaspoon, then finely grate the flesh. Fresh ginger is best kept in the freezer and can be grated from frozen.

GREEN BEANS & PEAS include French beans, flat beans, runner beans, broad beans, garden peas, sugar snaps and mangetout. Some will need trimming or podding, but these are an easy way to add a flash of green to any meal and require only minimal cooking, if any. Some are real seasonal stars, while others are easily found all year round. All are best stored in the fridge. Don't feel shy about using frozen peas and broad beans; they are among the few fresh veg to freeze well and will save you prep time.

LEAFY GREENS that are not brassicas include chard, pak choi and spinach, and extend to wild garlic and nettle tops

when they're in season. These can all be wilted down as a side dish, or added to a dish or stir-fry for the final few minutes. Spinach will overcook quickly, so always add it at the very last minute. The chard stalks and leaves are best cooked separately as the stalks take longer to cook. The tender crunch of the pak choi stalks are part of their charm, so can be cooked alongside their leaves.

LEMONGRASS is citrussy and fragrant, an essential ingredient in Southeast Asian cookery. It is very fibrous and woody, so unless you are blitzing it into a paste with other ingredients, the best way to release the flavour is to bash it with a rolling pin. Add it to the dish to infuse its flavour and remove it before serving.

MUSHROOMS Button, chestnut, Portobello and shiitake are the most common, but many more wild and delectable varieties are available at the right time of year. The flavour is dark and savoury, which adds depth as well and texture to a dish. You can slice and fry them or roast them whole. Best kept covered and in the fridge.

NUTS AND SEEDS can add body and bulk to a dish, or crunch and texture to a salad, and even be used as a garnish. Their flavour can be enhanced by lightly toasting them in a moderate oven or tossing them in a dry frying pan over a steady medium heat. Keep a careful eye on them, as they will become bitter if burnt. Most nuts and seeds can be blended into a spreadable paste or butter. Try to buy your nuts and seeds in small amounts and with a long use-by date on the pack, as their natural oil content can become rancid and bitter with age, so it doesn't make sense to store them in bulk. Cashews and pecans can be soaked overnight and blended to make fantastic plant-based creams. You'll notice that walnuts and flaxseeds are used in several of our recipes. They are both important sources of plant-based omega-3 fatty acids that can be added to pretty much any dish.

ONIONS AND ALLIUMS include white onions, red onions, shallots, spring onions, leeks and garlic. They all have a pungent kick when raw, but soften and sweeten beautifully when cooked. Allow onions at least ten minutes to soften and mellow before adding other

ingredients. This avoids the flavour of half-cooked onions dominating the dish. Keep your leeks and spring onions in the fridge; the rest are happy somewhere cool and dark.

PEPPERS, also known as sweet peppers, are generally bell-shaped, but long tapered varieties are increasingly common, as are 'baby' varieties. They can be used raw, but soften and mellow when slowly cooked. Roasting deepens their flavour, but the skin and seeds must be removed before using the flesh. You can buy excellent jars of pre-roasted peppers in most supermarkets.

RADISHES have a crunchy bite and a mild, peppery heat. Almost always used raw, they can be lightly braised or added to a stir fry. If the tops look good, they can be cooked too. Use within days of buying.

RED AND BLACK BEANS include kidney beans, black beans and black-eyed beans, which have a slightly firmer texture than white beans and are almost exclusively used in spicy cuisines, from Mexican chillies to Indian curries, and the spicy stews of the southern USA. As with the other beans, you can soak and cook them, or buy then canned for convenience.

ROOT VEGETABLES include potatoes, carrots, beetroots, parsnips and celeriac. They can all be roasted, boiled, steamed, braised, fried and mashed/puréed. Apart from potatoes, they can also be used raw. They don't need to be kept refrigerated, just somewhere dark and cool. Keep your fridge space free for the greener and more perishable veg.

SALAD LEAVES cover a multitude, including all varieties of lettuce, radicchio, rocket, watercress and pea shoots. Try to make your green salads interesting and varied, as far from plain old iceberg as you can get! A good mix of flavours is ideal. Some are very distinct, such as rocket (peppery), radicchio (bitter) and romaine (mild but crunchy), but will balance each other out nicely if combined. Some will even take well to being cooked – little gem, radicchio and watercress in particular.

SOYBEANS (also known as edamame beans) are a keystone of your plant-based diet. You can buy them fresh or frozen, and in the form of tofu and tempeh. All are now widely available in supermarkets and health food stores, as well as through online retailers, many of whom offer next-day delivery.

SPICES are essential, but generally bought in small amounts. However, the more you cook from scratch, the faster you'll get through them. The list below covers the spices used in this book, and for ease of explanation, I have grouped them by their general characteristics.

Aromatic/fragrant spices have distinct and complex flavours that are unmistakable. A little often goes a long way. Generally, they are ground to a powder, although some are used in seed form. Think cardamom, caraway, coriander, fennel seed, garam masala (spice mix), saffron and star anise.

Dominant spices such as cayenne, chilli powder, cloves and smoked paprika can easily overpower the other flavours in a dish. Use them in small amounts.

Earthy spices have comforting, well-rounded flavours that act as great bass notes in both sweet and savoury dishes. They have a hint of Christmas and winter about them. Think allspice, cinnamon, cumin, ginger, nutmeg, vanilla (extract) and turmeric.

SPLIT PEAS & LENTILS do not need soaking before being cooked. They'll benefit from a rinse, but you can add them straight to a dish and they'll absorb the liquid and plump up in 25–45 minutes, depending on the variety and how long they have been stored. Make sure they are well cooked and don't have a chalky bite to them. Handily, ready-cooked lentils, especially the dark Puy variety, are readily available to buy in cans and packets.

SPROUTED SEEDS AND BEANS are simply pulses, beans or seeds that have been soaked for a few days to promote sprouting. The most common are alfalfa, soy or mung beans, but a wide range of others is now available. The sprouting process can increase the availability of certain nutrients, including iron, zinc and vitamin C, and helps to develop a fresh, nutty taste and texture. Take care to follow the use-

by date so you get maximum benefit from the sprouts' high protein content, which spoils over time.

SQUASH range from the relatively soft cucumbers and courgettes to the heavy and solid butternut and autumnal squashes, such as kabocha and crown prince. The softer ones are easily sliced or peeled, can be eaten cooked or raw, and need keeping in the fridge. The tougher-skinned ones need peeling, cutting and deseeding before use – either roasted or simmered in a stew or curry. They'll keep for a week at room temperature.

SWEETCORN is best eaten fresh from the cob, but frozen is fine, and canned is also okay. Remove the husks, then cut off the kernels and use them in soups, stews and chowders, or boil the cobs whole and gnaw away at them. If barbecuing, leave the husks on and soak the cobs in water for at least 30 minutes before cooking. Place on the hot rack and cook until the husks are burnt, but the inside is perfectly cooked. Use fresh corn as soon as possible after buying.

TAHINI is a paste made from sesame seeds and lends itself to dressings and dips. You'll see it in several of our recipes.

TEMPEH is made from cooked soybeans that have been packed into solid blocks and slightly fermented. The fermentation gives it a distinct savoury flavour, but it is neutral enough to be marinated and easily flavoured. It holds its shape well and can be sliced or diced for roasting of frying.

TOFU is made from soya bean curds, which are pressed into blocks. It has a neutral flavour, so will carry any amount of saucing and spicing. Various textures are available: silken tofu is soft, creamy and breaks up or blends easily, while firm and extra-firm tofu can be diced or sliced and will marinate well. Firmer varieties can also be roasted, seared or barbecued without breaking up.

TOMATOES are noticeably better when locally grown and in season, and there are plenty of glorious shapes and colours available. Cold storage dulls the flavour, so store them at room

temperature and use when perfectly ripe. For many meals you'll use tomatoes canned and chopped, or as passata if making a sauce.

WHITE BEANS include haricot, cannellini, borlotti and butter beans. Despite their different colours, they all have the same kind of mild white flesh and soft skins when cooked. You can buy them dried or ready-cooked. They are interchangeable in the recipes but give them a bit of extra time to soak up all the surrounding flavours if added to a soup or stew.

WHOLEGRAINS are unrefined, which means they retain their fibre-packed bran, endosperm and germ layers, and thus offer maximum nutrition. They include barley, brown rice, bulgur, farro, freekeh, oats, polenta, quinoa, rye, spelt, wholemeal wheat flour and wild rice. Some wholegrains are processed into flours or are rolled or cracked to make them easier to cook or more suitable for specific dishes. If buying these products, always check the packet to ensure you're getting the whole grain, take care to follow the use-by date.

As a rule, wholegrains cook by absorbing liquid and plumping up. This process speeds up when they have been broken down. If you flavour the liquid in any way – with herbs, spices or stock, for example – the grains will absorb that flavouring too, which is why they make great additions to stews and braises. Some grains benefit from rinsing or soaking before use, and this is highlighted where required in the recipes. Some also take kindly to being lightly toasted in a dry pan before liquid is added; toasting can enhance the flavour, adding extra nuttiness and complexity.

When cooking and cooling grains to reheat later, take care to cool them as fast and thoroughly as you can, and then to store them in the fridge, just as you would beans and pulses. Food poisoning is all too common from rice that has been left at room temperature and then reheated.

ZUCCHINI is the American word for courgettes!

RECOMMENDED RESOURCES

Now that you've joined the Plant-based Diet Revolution, you'll want to learn more recipes and continue your education on the benefits this healthier approach to food. Here are some of my favourite resources.

COOKBOOKS

I love cookbooks just as much as I love medical journals. If you're looking for more healthy plant-based meals to inspire you every day, here are a few of my favourites.

BOSH! Healthy Vegan by Henry Firth and Ian Theasby (HQ Publishing, 2019)
The boys at BOSH TV have previously been known for making plant-based versions of some of the most indulgent dishes around, but Ian and Henry's healthiest cookbook to date is fully loaded with whole-food, plant-based goodness. This one is a firm favourite at our house.

Deliciously Ella: The Plant-based Cookbook by Ella Mills (Yellow Kite, 2018)
Having successfully improved her own health through a plant-based diet, Ella Mills shares the delicious recipes that she, her family and her customers continue to enjoy each day. As well as beautiful unfussy dishes, this book contains a fascinating and honest account of Ella's personal journey from vegan blogger to plant-based superstar.

No Meat Athlete Cookbook by Matt Frazier and Stephanie Romine (The Experiment, 2017)
Not just for the athlete in your life, this cookbook has dozens of easy to prepare meals that will satisfy all appetites. Conveniently, each recipe comes with a gluten-free or no-oil version for those who might need it.

The Bluezones Kitchen: 100 recipes to live to 100 by Dan Buettner (Penguin Random House, 2020)
Building on decades of research, longevity guru Dan Buettner gathered 100 beautiful recipes from the world's Blue Zones, home to the healthiest and happiest communities in the world. Its no surprise that all 100 recipes are made with wholefoods and are completely plant-based.

The Happy Pear: Recipes for Happiness by Stephen and David Flynn, (Penguin Ireland, 2018)
Steve and Dave know their way around a healthy kitchen! This book promises 'delicious, easy veggie food to be at your best' – and it delivers. You'll also find bonus chapters on the fundamentals of happiness and how to do a hand-stand!

The How Not to Die Cookbook by Michael Greger MD (Bluebird Publishing, 2018)
The team at nutritionfacts.org produced these recipes using only the very healthiest of ingredients. This is the perfect cookbook to help you continue your plant-based diet revolution.

The Vegiterranean Diet: The New and Improved Mediterranean Eating Plan by Julieanna Hever MS, RD, CPT (Da Capo Lifelong Books, 2015)
In this beautifully illustrated cookbook, renowned dietitian and author Julieanna Hever brings you satisfying meals that combine the best of plant-based and Mediterranean cooking.

WEBSITES

There are an infinite number of websites on human health and nutrition available, but not all can be trusted. Here are some of my recommended online resources.

bda.co.uk
The homepage of the British Dietetic Association, the professional body for dietitians in Britain. A leading resource on all matters related to healthy eating.

eatright.org
The American Academy of Nutrition and Dietetics is the largest professional body for registered dietitians in the world. Their website includes some wonderful plant-based recipes.

netflix.com
The world's number one provider of streamed TV and film entertainment is home to several compelling documentaries on the benefits of a healthier approach to food. If you or a friend are subscribers, why not make up a batch of Spicy tofu rolls (page 102) and enjoy *The Game Changers, What the Health,* or *Forks Over Knives* tonight?

nutritionfacts.org
The educational resources found at the homepage of Dr Michael Greger and his team of researchers are second to none.

pbhp.uk
I'm proud to be an ambassador and founding member of Plant-Based Health Professionals UK, a not-for profit group that was established to educate medical professionals, members of the public and policy-makers on the benefits of a whole-food, plant-based diet.

pcrm.org
The Physicians' Committee for Responsible Medicine has been educating US health professionals on the benefits of plant-based eating for decades. Their homepage has dozens of resources that come highly recommended.

vegansociety.com
The UK's Vegan Society has been around for 75 years. Their homepage is a great resource for all things plant-based, including Incredibly useful Information leaflets on planning a health diet at all ages.

PODCASTS

My favourite way to learn about what's current in the world of nutritional science.

The Exam Room Podcast
A fun and informative show from the doctors and nutrition experts at the Physicians' Committee for Responsible Medicine.

The Ian Cramer Podcast
Each week host Ian Cramer picks the brains of thought leaders within the realm of lifestyle medicine.

The Plant Proof Podcast
With a master's degree in nutrition, host Simon Hill knows exactly what questions to ask. If you love delving into the science, this podcast is for you.

The Rich Roll Podcast
Rich Roll has been recognised as one of the fittest men on the planet, pushing the limits of physical endurance, all while powered by plants.
His podcast brings you long-form interviews with 'the world's brightest and most thought-provoking thought leaders designed to educate, inspire and empower you to unleash your best, most authentic self'. Enjoy!

INDEX

Note: page numbers in *italics* refer to photographs.

A

advanced glycosylation end products 53
alcohol consumption 39
algae 212
almond 72, 111, 192
    barbecued nectarine & almonds 178, *179*
Alzheimer's disease 55
American Academy of Nutrition and
    Dietetics 10, 19
American Dietetic Association 213–14
American Gut Project 30, 31
anaphylaxis 213
anti-inflammatory diets 18, 33–4, 46, 50, 53,
    60, 212–13
antibiotics 33
antioxidants 15, 33
apple 74, 75, 116
    apple & apricot crumble *182*, 183
    apple & blackberry ice lollies 187, *188*
    stewed apples & cinnamon 69
apricot
    apple & apricot crumble *182*, 183
    dried apricot 149, 183
    roasted stone fruits *67*, 68
arachidonic acid (AA) 53
arthritis 31, 33
artichoke 215
    stuffed peppers with artichokes, fennel
    & farro 138, *139*
asparagus 76, 108, 140, 215
atherosclerosis 40, 42, 46, 55
athletes 50
aubergine 134, 150, 215
    miso aubergines with tofu fried rice
    168, 169
avocado 164, 215
    avocado on toast with four twists 118–19,
    120–1

B

banana 75, 184
    banana pecan ice cream 186, *189*
    nut butter & banana on toast 72, *73*
    quick banana & blueberry pancakes
    80, *81*
basal metabolic rate 45
batch cooking 200
bean(s) 18–19, 108, 150, 201, 212, 214–17

pakora bean burgers with raita & sweet
    potato chips 162, *163*
see also black bean; edamame beans;
    green bean; kidney bean; white bean
beetroot 116
    beetroot, sauerkraut & watercress
    sandwich 100, *101*
berries 190
    berry oat smoothie 74
    summer berries 69
    see also specific berries
black bean 91, 216
    chocolate beanie brownies 184, *185*
    guacamole toast with popped beans
    119, *121*
    loaded sweet potato with jerk black
    beans & peppers 87, *89*
blackberry
    apple & blackberry ice lollies 187, *188*
    quinoa porridge with blackberries &
    pistachios 64, *66*
blood pressure 38, 42, 45, 56, 196, 199
blood sugar levels 46, 199
blood vessels 55
blueberry, quick banana & blueberry
    pancakes 80, *81*
body, healthy 44–51
body mass index (BMI) 197
body weight 39
    see also obesity; overweight; weight
    gain; weight loss
bone health 213
bowel cancer 20, 24, 35–6
brain 55
brassicas 215
bread 100, 102, 150, 190
    brown soda bread *70*, 71
    easy wholegrain breads *70*, 71
    rye bread porridge with orange &
    prunes 65
    wholemeal flatbreads 133, *153*
    see also toast
breakfasts 62–83, 203, 205, 207, 209
breastfeeding 214
broth, squash & lemongrass noodle broth
    136, *137*
brownies, chocolate beanie brownies 184,
    185
buckwheat, spelt & buckwheat pancakes 80
bulgur wheat, tahini cauliflower with Greek
    bulgur wheat 170, *171*

burgers, pakora bean burgers with raita &
    sweet potato chips 162, *163*

C

cabbage 104, 116
    rosti pie with braised cabbage & peas
    126, 127
cacao nibs 184, 186
    cherry cacao bars 192
cacao powder 72, 74, 180, 184, 186
caffeine 213
calcium 17, 25, 196, 213
calorie-burning 45
calorie-counting 196
calorie-dense food 10, 17
cancer 12, 20, 23–5, 33, 35–6, 44, 56, 213
canned food 201
caper(s) 92, 138
carbohydrates 14, 23, 45
    complex 14, 17, 30
    simple 14
    whole 23
carcinogens 36
cardiovascular disease 23, 38, 40, 56, 213
carrot 96, 102, 104, 124, 127, 144, 162
    carrot cake bites 180, *181*
cashew nut
    brown rice porridge with coconut,
    cashew & mango 65
    cashew cream 190
cauliflower 158
    cauliflower, butter bean & chard dahl
    154, *155*
    tahini cauliflower with Greek bulgur
    wheat 170, *171*
celeriac 127, 158
celery 104, 108, 111–12, 124, 127, 144, 158, 215
chard
    cauliflower, butter bean & chard dahl
    154, *155*
    loaded sweet potato with sweetcorn &
    chard 87, *89*
cherry cacao bars 192, *193*
chicken 10
chickpea(s) 90, 100, 107, 111, 152, 215
    loaded sweet potato with chickpea
    tabbouleh 86, *88*
    plant-powered stew with braised
    hickpeas & couscous 134, *135*
children 213–14
chilli (dish), one-pot chilli bowl 164, *165*

chips, pakora bean burgers with raita &
sweet potato chips 162, *163*
chocolate
chocolate beanie brownies 184, *185*
chocolate chip ice cream 186
dreamy hot chocolate 180, *181*
cholesterol 40–2, 45, 48, 196–7
choline-containing foods 17
coconut flakes, barbecued mango &
coconut 178, *179*
coconut milk 75, 137, 152
brown rice porridge with coconut,
cashew & mango 65
coeliac disease 212–13
coffee 74, 213
Complete Health Improvement Programme
45
compotes 68–9
Coprococcus 53
courgette 96, 104, 140, 150, 217
farinata with courgettes, tomatoes &
capers 92, *95*
sticky tofu, courgettes, greens & kimchi
146, *147*
couscous 134
plant-powered stew with braised
chickpeas & couscous 134, *135*
COVID-19 (coronavirus pandemic) 56
cows' milk 25, 213
Crohn's disease 9, 33, 34
crumble, apple & apricot crumble *182*, 183
cucumber 86, 100, 130, 162, 170
curry, sweet potato massaman curry 152, *153*

D

dairy foods 12, 25, 33, 39
date(s) 180, 184
dementia 55
depression 33, 52–3
dhal, cauliflower, butter bean & chard dahl
154, 155
diabetes 20, 23
type 1 29
type 2 10, 12, 24, 30–1, 33, 35, 46–8, 50, 52,
56, 196, 199
Diehl, Hans 45
dietary diversity 22, 30–1, 33, 42
dinners 122–73, 203, 205, 207, 209
dips, sweet tahini dip 175, 176
doctor's letters 199
dressings 96, 104, 114, 130, 132, 200
drinks 18, 39, 201
dumplings, winter barley stew with Irish
stout & herby dumplings 144, *145*

E

EAT-*Lancet* report 10
eating, mindful 51
eating out 198
edamame beans 140, 212, 216–17
egg 10
EpiPens 213
Esselstyn, Caldwell, Jr 40

F

falafel, speedy falafels & more *106*, 107
farinata, savoury farinata 92–3, *92–3*
farls, spicy baked beans & sweet potato
farl 78, *79*
farro, stuffed peppers with artichokes,
fennel & farro 138, *139*
fat cells 44
fats 14, 17
fatty liver disease 44, 48
Feacalibacterium 53
fennel 116, 215
Spanish rice with fennel, tomato &
olives 157
stuffed peppers with artichokes, fennel
& farro 138, *139*
fermentation 30
fermented foods 37
fibre 30, 35–6, 59, 196, 198
fibre-deficient gut 35–6
fish 10
'five-a-day' 13
flatbreads, wholemeal flatbreads 133, *133*
FODMAPs 214
food diaries 12
freekeh, squash & olive tagine with freekeh
148, 149
French bean 152, 156
frozen foods 201
fruit 12, 20, 215
barbecued fruit 178, *179*
the big fruit bowl with sweet tahini dip
175, 176
and diabetes 46
dried 104, 132, 149, 183, 201, 215
portion sizes 13
recommended intake 18, 19
roasted stone fruits *67*, 68
shopping lists 202, 204, 206, 208
see also specific fruits
frying, without oil 60

G

gastroenterology 7, 9
genes 44, 55

ginger 216
pears & ginger 69
gluten 59, 212–13
goal-setting 196
gooseberry 68
goulash hotpot 160, *161*
gratin, roasting tray ratatouille gratin 150,
151
gravy, epic nut roast with onion miso gravy
166, *167*
green bean 152, 216
Cajun beans & greens 156
farinata with masala green beans, peas
& spring onions 93, *94*
greenhouse gas emissions 20
guacamole toast with popped beans 119,
120
gut bacteria 29–37, 47–8, 53, 198, 214
gut-brain connection 53

H

happiness effect 52–3
hash, spring tofu hash 76, *77*
health
goals for 196
prescriptions for 22–6
healthy diets 10
Healthy Eating Index (HEI) 12
heart attack 38–41
heart disease 10, 12, 18, 20, 23–5, 30–1, 33,
39–42, 44–6, 56, 60, 197
heart health 38–43
herbs 18, 201, 202, 204, 206, 208, 215–16
Hippocrates 10
history taking 13
hotpot, goulash hotpot 160, *161*
hummus 90–1, 99
basic hummus 90, *90*
herby white bean hummus 90, *91*
mushroom & walnut hummus *90*, 91
Tex-Mex hummus *90*, 91
hyperglycaemia 46
hypertension 38, 42, 45, 56, 196, 199

I

ice cream
banana pecan ice cream 186, *189*
raspberry ripple ice cream 186
ice lollies
apple & blackberry ice lollies 187, *188*
strawberry mini milks 187, *188*
inflammation 44
chronic 33–4, 44, 48, 53, 55, 212
gut 9, 32, 34, 48, 212

see also anti-inflammatory diets
inflammatory bowel disease 24, 26
insulin resistance 46
iron 17, 196, 213
irritable bowel syndrome (IBS) 35, 196

J
junk food 10, 22, 32

K
kale 158, 172
    corn & squash spelt risotto with black
        kale 128, 129
    squash & raw kale quinoa salad 114, 115
kedgeree, baked kedgeree with roast
    tomatoes, mushrooms & spinach 82, 83
kidney bean 164
    Cajun beans & greens 156
kimchi 37
sticky tofu, courgettes, greens & kimchi
    146, 147
koftas, speedy koftas 107

L
'leaky gut' syndrome 30, 32
lectins 214
legumes 12, 20, 39, 212, 215
lemongrass 216
lentil(s) 91, 107, 127, 166, 172, 217
    cauliflower, butter bean & chard dahl
        155
    Lebanese lentil & tahini pittas 132–3
    spicy parsnip & lentil winter soup 112,
        113
lettuce 130
    MLT sandwich 98, 99
low-carb diets 23
low-fibre diets 36
lunches 51, 84–121, 203, 205, 207, 209

M
magnesium-containing foods 17
Magnetic Resonance Imaging (MRI) 35
mango 75
    barbecued mango & coconut 178, 179
    brown rice porridge with coconut,
        cashew & mango 65
    mango sorbet 187, 189
    pineapple or mango 69
marinades 146, 170
meal plans 200–9
meat 12, 46, 56
    processed 20, 39
    red 10, 20, 33, 35, 39

meat alternatives 212
medications 196, 199
Mediterranean diet 12, 20, 52–3
mental health 52–5
metabolic syndrome 48
microbiome 29–37, 47–8, 53, 198, 214
milk 25, 213
mindful eating 51
minerals 15
    see also specific minerals
minestrone, chunky minestrone 108, 109
miso 60
    epic nut roast with onion miso gravy
        166, 167
    miso aubergines with tofu fried rice
        168, 169
    tempeh miso stir-fry 142, 143
mocha oat smoothie 74
multivitamins, VEG-1 24, 26
mushroom 119, 124, 127, 137, 142, 144, 166,
    172, 216
    baked kedgeree with roast tomatoes,
        mushrooms & spinach 82, 83
    farinata with mushrooms, spinach,
        garlic & chilli 93, 94
    MLT sandwich 98, 99
    mushroom & walnut hummus 90, 91

N
nature, spending time in 33
nectarine
    barbecued nectarine & almonds 178, 179
    roasted stone fruits 67, 68
non-coeliac wheat sensitivity 213
noodle(s) 142
    fiery noodle salad 96, 97
    squash & lemongrass noodle broth
        136, 137
nutrients 14–17
nut(s) 18–20, 39, 116, 201, 216
    epic nut roast with onion miso gravy
        166, 167
    nut butter & banana on toast 72, 73

O
oat(s) 180, 183, 192
    breakfast oat smoothies 74, 75
    oat bread 71
    simple oat porridge 64
obesity 10, 12, 30–1, 33–4, 36, 41, 44–6, 48, 56
'obesogenic environment' 44, 51
oils 14, 201
    added 12, 18, 60
olive 134, 138, 170

Spanish rice with fennel, tomato &
    olives 157
squash & olive tagine with freekeh 148,
    149
olive oil 18, 20, 60
omega-3 fatty acids 17, 212
omega-6 fatty acids 17
omnivores 12
onion 216
    epic nut roast with onion miso gravy
        166, 167
orange, rye bread porridge with orange &
    prunes 65
organic produce 21
overweight 41, 45
    see also obesity

P
pak choi 96, 142, 146
pakora bean burgers with raita & sweet
    potato chips 162, 163
pancakes
    quick banana & blueberry pancakes
        80, 81
    spelt & buckwheat pancakes 80
Parkinson's disease 31
parsnip 104, 158
    spicy parsnip & lentil winter soup 112,
        113
passata 78, 134
pasta
    chunky minestrone 108
    summer veg & white bean pasta 140, 141
peach, roasted stone fruits 67, 68
peanut 104, 152
peanut butter 64, 80, 87, 96, 102, 192
pear 104
    pears & ginger 69
pearl barley, winter barley stew with Irish
    stout & herby dumplings 144, 145
pea(s) 108, 140, 157, 169, 216
    farinata with masala green beans, peas
        & spring onions 93, 94
    rosti pie with braised cabbage & peas
        126, 127
pecan, banana pecan ice cream 186, 189
pepper 134, 150, 156, 160, 164, 216
    loaded sweet potato with jerk black
        beans & peppers 87, 89
    Spanish red pepper soup 110, 111
    stuffed peppers with artichokes, fennel
        & farro 138, 139
pescatarians 12
pesticides 21

pesto, avocado pesto toast with tomatoes 118, *121*

phosphorus-containing foods 17

physical exercise 33, 39, 51

phytonutrients 15

pies, rosti pie with braised cabbage & peas *126, 127*

pilaf, winter pilaf 158, *159*

pine nut(s) 91, 118

pineapple or mango 69

pistachio, quinoa porridge with blackberries & pistachios 64, *66*

pittas, Lebanese lentil & tahini pittas 132–3

plum, spiced plums 68

polenta, hearty Bolognese with squash & rosemary polenta 124, *125*

porridge

    brown rice porridge with coconut, cashew & mango 65

    quinoa porridge with blackberries & pistachios 64, *66*

    rye bread porridge with orange & prunes 65

    simple oat porridge 64

portion sizes 202

potassium-containing foods 17

potato 76, 108, 127, 144, 160

pre-diabetes 34

prebiotics 29

pregnancy 214

preserves 201

Prevotella 31

pro-inflammatory substances 36, 43–4, 46, 48, 214

probiotics 29, 53

processed foods 12, 20, 22, 39, 42

protein 10, 14, 17, 24, 40, 50, 59, 196

prune, rye bread porridge with orange & prunes 65

pulses 201

pumpkin seed 128, 158, 192

Q

quinoa 164, 166

    quinoa porridge with blackberries & pistachios 64, *66*

    squash & raw kale quinoa salad 114, *115*

R

radish 96, 102, 104, 216

    avocado toast with radish & sprouted seeds 118, *120*

raita, pakora bean burgers with raita & sweet potato chips 162, *163*

Ramage, Andy *42*

raspberry ripple ice cream 186

ratatouille, roasting tray ratatouille gratin 150, *151*

refrigerating food 200

reheating food 200

rhubarb 68

rice 82, 146, 152, 156

    brown rice porridge with coconut, cashew & mango 65

    miso aubergines with tofu fried rice *168, 169*

    Spanish rice with fennel, tomato & olives 157

    wild rice super salad 116, *117*

    winter pilaf 158, *159*

risotto, corn & squash spelt risotto with black kale 128, *129*

rosti pie with braised cabbage & peas *126, 127*

rye bread porridge with orange & prunes 65

S

salads 216

    crispy tofu tacos & chopped salsa salad 130, *131*

    fiery noodle salad 96, *97*

    squash & raw kale quinoa salad 114, *115*

    wild rice super salad 116, *117*

salt *42*, 60

sandwiches

    beetroot, sauerkraut & watercress sandwich 100, *101*

    MLT sandwich 98, *99*

sauerkraut 37

    beetroot, sauerkraut & watercress sandwich 100, *101*

seasoning 18, 60

seeds 18, 19, 20, 201, 216

selenium-containing foods 17

Seventh Day Adventists 39

shopping lists 51, 200, 202, 204, 206, 208

short-chain fatty acids (SCFAs) 30, 37, 47, 53

slaws, three fresh slaws 104, *105*

sleep 33

smoking 39

smoothies, breakfast oat smoothies 74, *75*

snacks 203, 205, 207, 209

social support 197

sorbet, mango sorbet 187, *189*

soup

    chunky minestrone 108, *109*

    Spanish red pepper soup 110, *111*

spicy parsnip & lentil winter soup 112, *113*

South-West Plant-based Diet Challenge 41

soy sauce 60

soya beans 140, 212, 216–17

spelt

    corn & squash spelt risotto with black kale 128, *129*

    spelt & buckwheat pancakes 80

spices 18, 201, 217

spinach 134, 156–7

    baked kedgeree with roast tomatoes, mushrooms & spinach 82, *83*

    farinata with mushrooms, spinach, garlic & chilli 93, *94*

split pea (s) 217

spring onion, farinata with masala green beans, peas & spring onions 93, *94*

sprouted seeds 96, 104, 142

    avocado toast with radish & sprouted seeds 118, *120*

    sprouted seeds and beans 217

squash 166, 172, 217

    corn & squash spelt risotto with black kale 128, *129*

    hearty Bolognese with squash & rosemary polenta 124, *125*

    squash & lemongrass noodle broth *136, 137*

    squash & olive tagine with freekeh 148, *149*

    squash & raw kale quinoa salad 114, *115*

Standard Western Diet 10, 12, 30–1, 35–6, 44, 48, 56

stew

    winter barley stew with Irish stout & herby dumplings 144, *145*

    see also tagine

stir-fries, tempeh miso stir-fry 142, *143*

stock, vegetable stock 60

storage space 197

store-cupboard essentials 201, 202, 204, 206, 208

storing food 200

strawberry

    barbecued strawberry & balsamic 178, *179*

    strawberry mini milks 187, *188*

stroke 12, 20, 33, 38, 40–2, 44, 46, 197, 213

sugar 14, 18, 25

summer pudding, glorious summer pudding 190, *191*

sunlight 26

superfoods 20

swede 144

sweet potato
    loaded sweet potatoes 86–7, 88–9
    pakora bean burgers with raita & sweet
        potato chips 162, *163*
    spicy baked beans & sweet potato farl
        78, *79*
    sweet potato massaman curry 152, *153*
sweet treats 25, 174–93, 203, 205, 207, 209
sweetcorn 156, 217
    corn & squash spelt risotto with black
        kale 128, *129*
    loaded sweet potato with sweetcorn &
        chard 87, *89*

T
tabbouleh, loaded sweet potato with
    chickpea tabbouleh 86, *88*
tacos, crispy tofu tacos & chopped salsa
    salad 130, *131*
tagine, squash & olive tagine with freekeh
    148, *149*
tahini 90, 169, 170, 217
    the big fruit bowl with sweet tahini dip
        175, 176
    Lebanese lentil & tahini pittas 132–3
    tahini cauliflower with Greek bulgur
        wheat 170, *171*
tempeh 124, 212, 217
    autumn roasting tray tempeh 172
    tempeh miso stir-fry 142, *143*
time management 197
toast
    avocado on toast with four twists 118–19,
        120–1
    nut butter & banana on toast 72, *73*
tofu 212, 217
    crispy tofu tacos & chopped salsa salad
        130, *131*
    miso aubergines with tofu fried rice
        168, 169
    spicy tofu rolls 102, *103*
    spring tofu hash 76, *77*
    sticky tofu, courgettes, greens & kimchi
        146, *147*
tomato 86–7, 108, 111–12, 124, 134, 138, 150,
    155–6, 160, 164, 170, 217
    avocado pesto toast with tomatoes 118,
        121
    baked kedgeree with roast tomatoes,
        mushrooms & spinach 82, *83*
    crispy tofu tacos & chopped salsa salad
        130, *131*
    farinata with courgettes, tomatoes &
        capers 92, *95*

MLT sandwich *98*, 99
    Spanish rice with fennel, tomato &
        olives 157

U
ulcerative colitis 34

V
vegan diet 12, 50, 214
vegan poop transplant 31
vegetable stock 60
vegetables 12, 20, 39
    and diabetes 46
    diversity of 22, 30, 33, 42
    portion sizes 13
    preparation 200
    recommended intake 18, 19
    shopping lists 202, 204, 206, 208
vegetarian diet 12, 20
vitamin A 17
vitamin B12 24
vitamin B group 17, 24
vitamin C 17, 213
vitamin D 24, 26, 213
vitamin E 17
vitamin K 17
vitamins 15, 17, 24, 26, 213

W
walnut 72, 116, 158, 166, 172, 180
    mushroom & walnut hummus 90, 91
water-containing foods 17
watercress, beetroot, sauerkraut &
    watercress sandwich 100, *101*
watermelon, barbecued watermelon &
    mint 178, *179*
weight gain 44
weight loss 42, 45, 48, 197
wheat allergy 213
white bean 217
    cauliflower, butter bean & chard dahl
        154, 155
    herby white bean hummus 90, 91
    spicy baked beans & sweet potato farl
        78, *79*
    summer veg & white bean pasta 140, *141*
whole-food plant-based approach 14–21
wholegrains 12, 20, 23, 35, 39, 201, 212–14,
    217
    easy wholegrain breads *70*, 71
    portion sizes 13
    recommended intake 18, 19
World Health Organization (WHO) 36, 213

Y
yogurt, soya 162, 176

Z
zinc-containing foods 17
zoonotic diseases 56
zucchini 217

ACKNOWLEDGMENTS

Thank you to Hannah, for being the most inspiring person that I've ever met and for choosing to be my wife. To Rebecca, Naomi and Ethan, thank you for keeping us smiling and for understanding why sometimes your Dad still has work to do when he gets home. Thank you to my parents, Noel and Norma Desmond, for raising me to appreciate the true value of education, and to my in-laws Ed and Hilary Shiels for your endless support. Thank you to my sister Claudine for blazing the plant-based trail.

Thank you to my good friend, collaborator and co-author Bob Andrew for turning nutritional science into delicious recipes and for the many hours-long conversations that we really should have recorded. A huge thanks to my dietitian colleagues, especially to Rosie Martin for her meticulous work analysing the recipes and meal plans and for every other project that we have worked on together. Thank you to Deborah Howland and Sarah Jones, for being incredible colleagues. Thank you to Sharon, Nina and Jaye for keeping me organised and (sort of) on schedule.

Thank you to Stephen and David Flynn, for your constant encouragement, good vibes and undeniable enthusiasm for helping people to eat more plants. Thank you to Fiona McBennett and the wonderful team at the Happy Pear. Thanks to Tara O'Sullivan for being the original catalyst and to Faith O'Grady for championing this project. I owe a huge debt of gratitude to Sophie Elletson, Emma Knight, Caitriona Horne, Isabel Gonzalez-Prendergast, Olivia Nightingall, Nicky Ross and everyone at Yellow Kite. Thank you to Dan Jones for your beautiful photography and to Louise Leffler for making these pages look amazing. Thank you to Ian Theasby, Henry Firth, Dale Pinnock and Andy Ramage for sharing your wisdom and experience with this first-time author.

Everyone needs their plant-based tribe! Thank you Wade, Les, Matt, Suze, Chloe and Steve for being ours. Thank you Les for introducing me to Bob and for convincing Wade to move to Devon. Chloe and Danny, thank you so much for reading and vastly improving the early drafts. Thank you to Dr Shireen Kassam and to all my friends and colleagues at Plant-based Health Professionals UK for your support and for all that you do. I hope that everyone who reads this book will also visit www.pbhp.uk to learn more about our movement.

Above all, thank you to my patients for starting me on this journey and for continuing to inspire me every day.